THE

BLACK WOMAN'S

HAIR BIBLE

THE

BLACK WOMAN'S

HAIR BIBLE

EVERYTHING YOU HAVE ALWAYS
WANTED TO KNOW ABOUT YOUR
HAIR BUT DIDN'T KNOW WHO TO ASK

WRITTEN BY
LISA C. JOHNSON

MIDWEST PUBLISHING COMPANY

To all black women who wish to achieve
healthy, beautiful hair.

How to Read this Book

This book is meant to be an all purpose guide to Black hair care. It is a compilation of the best hair care practices learned over the years from books, the internet, friends and personal experience with my own hair. You can read it from cover to cover or you can a pick a chapter you find interesting and start from there.

- Lisa C. Johnson

TABLE OF CONTENTS

HAIR 101 : THE BASICS OF BLACK HAIR 13

TRANSITIONING TO NATURAL HAIR 35

CHAPTER ONE

HAIR 101 : THE BASICS OF BLACK HAIR

You're probably thinking, "Hair 101? I didn't sign up for this class. I just want the tips, the tricks, the secrets. All the exciting stuff!" . I promise will get to that, but it would be a disservice to you to not go over the basics of Black hair. Knowing the basics will let you have a better understanding of why the tips and tricks work.

So, without further ado, let's get right into the anatomy of Black hair.

Hair Anatomy

What is Hair?

Your hair is made up mostly of two things — protein and water. The type of protein in your hair is called *keratin* and is also found in your eyes, nails and skin. Each hair strand has 3 layers — the cuticle, the cortex and the medulla.

Layers of a hair strand

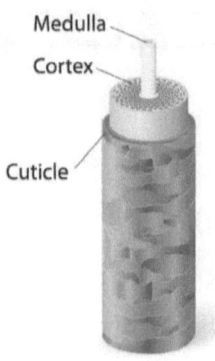

Figure 1. Illustration of a hair strand showing the medulla, cortex and cuticle.

The **cuticle** is the outermost layer of a hair strand. It has shingle like cells that overlap and work to *protect* the cortex. It is semi-transparent and *reflects* or *refracts* light to provide shine or sheen to your hair. The cuticle is responsible for maintaining moisture in the hair strand and a damaged cuticle will have trouble retaining moisture.

The cuticle can easily be damaged by chemical processes, heat, poor maintenance and constant manipulation.

The **cortex** is the middle layer of a hair strand. It is the cortex that provides hair with the majority of its weight (up to 90%) and gives it strength. The cortex also provides color to your hair through melanin — a pigment contained in the cortex. Using chemical relaxers and permanent hair coloring weaken the cortex.

The **medulla** is the innermost layer of a hair strand. The function of the medulla is not known and is found only in thicker hairs.

The Scalp

The scalp is skin. The scalp has three layers — the epidermis, the dermis and the hypodermis. The epidermis is the top layer, the dermis is the middle layer and the hypodermis is the bottom layer. Our hair grows out of the scalp and knowing what is happening underneath the scalp is key to understanding how to take care of your hair.

Cross section of the scalp

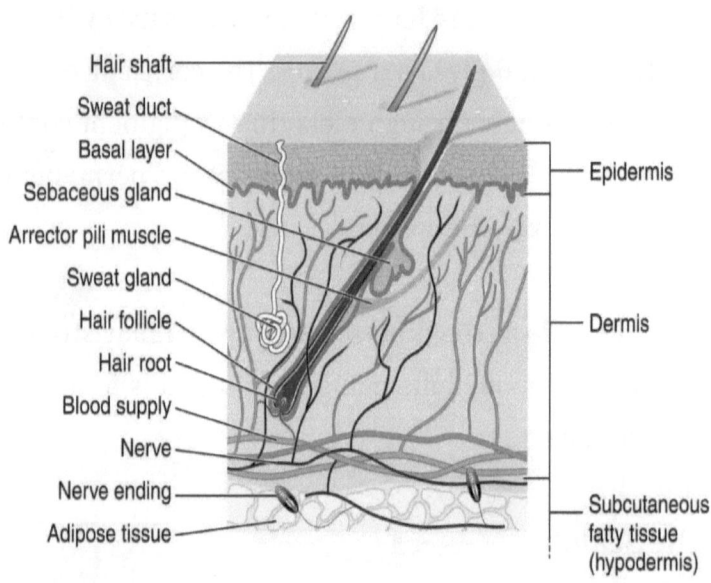

Figure 2. Illustration showing the epidermis ,dermis and hypodermis.

The **epidermis** is the top layer of the scalp and is the layer of the scalp that you can see and touch. When you scratch your scalp, you are scratching the epidermis. When you have dandruff, it is the epidermis that is shedding.

The **dermis** is the middle layer of the scalp, located between the epidermis which is above it and the hypodermis which is below it. The hair follicle, the sebaceous gland and the blood capillaries are all located in the dermis.

- **Hair follicle:** The hair follicle is responsible for producing hair. On average, there are about 100,000 hair follicles on your scalp.

- **Sebaceous gland:** The sebaceous gland is attached to the hair follicle and is responsible for producing *sebum* — a natural oil that lubricates the hair shaft and the scalp. Due to the kinky, coily nature of Black hair sebum has trouble travelling down the hair shaft. This makes our hair dry and not as well lubricated as Caucasian or Asian hair.

- **Blood capillaries / supply :** The blood capillaries are responsible for bringing nutrients to the hair follicle for hair growth.

Cross section of the hair bulb

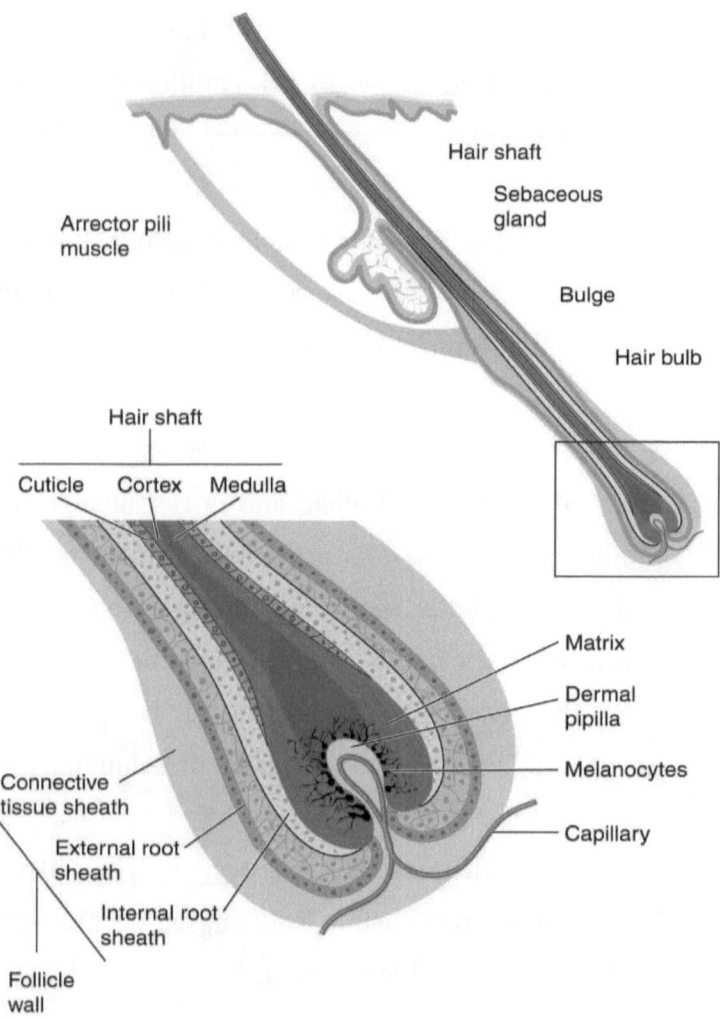

Figure 3. Illustration showing the hair bulb

The **hypodermis** is the bottom layer of the scalp. The hypodermis mainly consists of fat cells and nerve endings.

Hair Properties and Characteristics

Will now go over the properties and characteristics of your hair.

Hair Bonds

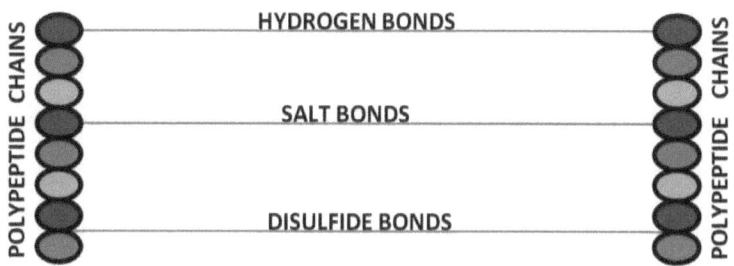

Figure 4. Illustration of hair bonds

Inside the cortex of each hair strand, there are long chains of amino acids. Amino acids are the building blocks of your hair. These amino acids are bound together by peptide bonds. When the amino acids are linked together to form a chain, they are called *polypeptide chains*.

Polypeptide chains are held together by side bonds.

Side bonds are responsible for the strength of your hair. Whenever heat or a chemical relaxer is applied to your hair, the side bonds are being broken down which weakens the hair.

The 3 different side bonds are:

1) *Hydrogen bonds*
2) *Salt Bonds*
3) *Disulfide bonds*

Hydrogen bonds are the weakest side bond and can easily be broken by water or heat. For example, applying heat to your hair breaks down the hydrogen bonds allowing the hair to straighten.

Salt bonds are also weak and can be broken by strong acidic or alkaline solutions.

Disulfide bonds are the strongest side bond but can still be broken by chemicals. When you get your hair relaxed, the relaxer breaks down the disulfide bonds resulting in your hair becoming straight. Once disulfide bonds are broken they cannot be restored or repaired.

Hair Color

The color of your hair is determined by the pigment melanin. Melanin is found in the strands of your hair. The range of natural color for black women's hair is black to brown.

Hair Density

Hair density is how close to each other the hair strands on your head are. *It is unrelated to the texture of your hair.* Hair density is measured by the number of hairs per square inch of your scalp. (The average density is 2,200 hairs per square inch).

Hair Elasticity

Hair elasticity is the measure of how much a hair strand will stretch and return to its normal length, without breaking. Your hair elasticity can be high, normal or low. Knowing the elasticity of your hair is important because it lets you know if your hair is weak and prone to breakage.

Hair with low elasticity can easily break, while hair with normal to high elasticity is more resistant to breakage. The major reasons why your hair may have low elasticity is lack of moisture, heat damage or chemical processing. To determine the elasticity of your hair, you will need to perform a strand test.

Strand test

After washing your hair and it's still wet, take a strand of your hair. Stretch the hair strand for a few seconds. If it bounces back to its original length you have normal to high elasticity. If it breaks, you have low elasticity. Low elasticity hair is weak and more likely to break when combing or brushing. To improve the elasticity of your hair, keep your hair moisturized, limit chemical processing and include a protein conditioner in your regimen.

Hair pH

pH stands for "power of Hydrogen" , it is a measure of how acidic or alkali a solution or substance is. pH is measured on a scale that ranges from 0 to 14. A substance having a pH of below 7 is *acidic*, a substance above 7 is *alkaline* and a substance with a pH of 7 is *neutral*.

Healthy hair and scalp has a pH range between 4.5 and 5.5. At this pH range, fungi and bacteria are prevented from growing. Also at this range, the hair cuticles are kept closed keeping moisture in and providing shine to your hair. When you use a product that is highly alkaline (like a chemical relaxer) the cuticles are opened up and when you use a product that is highly acidic (like apple cider vinegar) the cuticles contract and close.

Knowing the pH of a product you use is important because products that are within or close to the 4.5 to 5.5 range will work best for your hair. If you don't already do so, start testing the pH of shampoos and conditioners you use. You can find pH test strips at your local drugstore or beauty supply store.

Hair Porosity

Hair porosity is the ability of your hair to absorb moisture. Porosity can be high, low or normal.

High porosity hair is hair that has been damaged by over processing. As a result it will let moisture in and out easily. To repair this damage, use of a protein treatment is recommended. In addition, thick butters (like Shea butter) are best when sealing in moisture in high porosity hair.

Low porosity hair is hair that has tightly compact cuticles due to genetics. Low porosity hair has difficulty absorbing moisture. With low porosity hair, avoid products with a low pH. Low pH products will close the cuticle even further. Occasional use of a baking soda shampoo wash is recommended for low porosity hair (baking soda has a high pH and lifts up the cuticle to allow moisture from either a conditioner or moisturizer into the hair strand).

Normal porosity hair is hair that has a slightly compact cuticle. It is able to absorb and retain moisture well. If you have normal porosity hair, be mindful not to over process your hair as this can lead to high porosity hair.

Testing Your Hair's Porosity

To test the porosity of your hair, simply take one strand of hair and place it in small bowl filled with water. If the hair strand immediately sinks to the bottom, you have *high porosity*. If the hair strand does not sink and continually floats at the top, you have *low porosity*. If the hair strand floats at the top for a few minutes and then gradually sinks to the bottom, you have *normal porosity*.

Hair Shape

The natural curl pattern of your hair is determined by the shape of the follicle. When the follicle is round in shape, your hair will be straight. When the follicle is elliptical in shape your hair will be kinky. When the follicle is oval your hair will be curly.

The Shape of the hair follicle

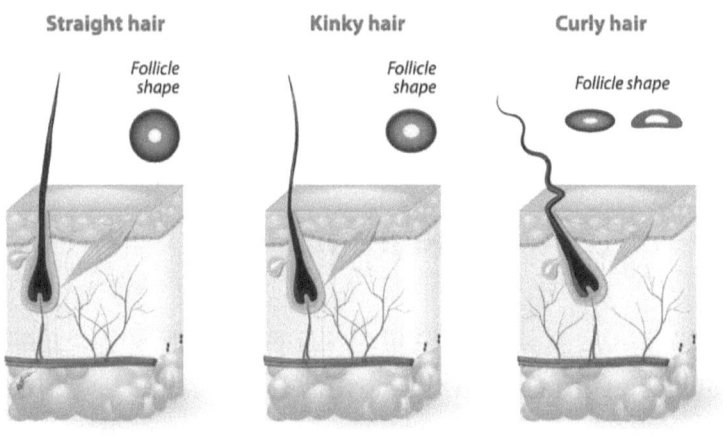

Figure 5 . Illustration showing shape of the hair follicle

Hair Shine

The shine of your hair is provided by the cuticle. A closed cuticle adds shine to the hair. Black hair does not have much shine due to its natural curl pattern. Our hair refracts light and needs oils or creams to increase its shine.

Hair Strength

The strength of your hair is determined by side bonds in the cortex. A proper balance between moisture and protein in the cortex provides your hair the maximum possible strength.

Hair Typing

Hair typing is any system that places hair into separate categories based on its texture. This can be difficult because one head of hair can have more than one texture. While hair typing systems are not scientific, they do allow women of similar hair types to share which products, styles and accessories work for them. The most commonly used hair typing system is the Andre Walker hair typing system .

The Andre Walker hair typing system classifies hair into one of 4 types. Type 1 is *straight*, Type 2 is *wavy*, Type 3 is *curly* and Type 4 is *kinky*. Most black women will be in the Type 4 category.

Common Myths About Black Hair Debunked

Myth 1: Black hair can't grow long

One of the biggest myths about black hair is that it can't grow long. This has been repeated so many times that many black women now believe that to be the truth. It is far from the truth. Others will say that you have to be "mixed with something" to have long hair — which again is not true — black women who properly maintain their hair and retain length can grow long hair.

Myth 2: Black hair is strong

Because of its texture, many women often assume their hair is strong. Black hair is actually the weakest of all human hair. The reason why it is the weakest is because each curl in a hair strand is a point of weakness and a potential breaking point.

In addition, because of the curl pattern, the natural oil sebum has more difficulty travelling down the hair shaft making our hair dry and more susceptible to breakage.

Myth 3: Split ends can be repaired by a product

Save your money, don't bother buying a product that promises it will repair your split ends. No product no matter what it promises can repair split ends. Once you have split ends, the only way to prevent them travelling up the hair shaft and causing more damage to your hair is to cut them off.

Myth 4: You need to grease your scalp

A common myth that has been passed down from generation to generation is that greasing your scalp helps your hair to grow. The petroleum and mineral oils contained in grease actually hinder hair growth by clogging the hair follicles on your scalp which can eventually lead to hair loss.

Myth 5: More expensive products are best for your

hair.

Most likely a myth started by companies that sell hair products. The truth is that the price of a hair product has no relation to how well it will work on your hair. What is more important than the price of a product is knowing the ingredients and what those ingredients do for your hair. Become knowledgeable about product ingredients and find products that contain ingredients that are best for your hair.

Myth 6: You should avoid water

Another myth that's just not true. Your hair needs moisture. Our hair is naturally dry and must be moisturized to keep it healthy and avoid breakage. Think of your hair as a plant that needs to be watered.

Myth 7: Trimming will make your hair grow

Trimming your hair does not make your hair grow. Your hair grows from the roots not the ends. Trimming your hair excessively actually makes it more difficult to get long hair. If you are constantly trimming your hair, how can your hair grow longer?

Trimming should only be done with reason. That reason should be to cut off split ends or when transitioning to natural hair to remove the relaxed ends.

Myth 8: Hair growth creams and pills work

Another popular myth is that hair growth creams and pills work. "Magic" hair growth creams and pills are popular because they provide hope. Hope that you can apply a cream to your scalp and then you will magically have longer hair.

Most of these growth creams actually contain ingredients that can damage your hair and impede hair growth. Growing hair is all about retaining length and reducing breakage. *There is no magic to it.*

Myth 9: There is one product that's out there that works for every woman's hair — you just have to find it.

This myth has turned a lot of women into product junkies continually searching for the holy grail of product that will solve all their hair problems. The truth is no one product will work for every black woman's hair. The reason is that hair is unique and how your hair responds to one product, is different to how someone else's hair responds to that same product.

Myth 10: Your hair grows faster when relaxed.

Your hair grows at the same rate whether its relaxed or natural. Relaxing your hair does not change your *natural rate of growth*. It might seem to be growing faster when you have it relaxed because it grows down your back, but it's growing at the same rate.

Myth 11: A dirty scalp will make your hair grow faster.

Another myth that has been passed down from generation to generation. A dirty scalp does not make your hair grow any faster and can actually have the opposite effect. Product build up can clog the pores, cause dandruff and an itchy scalp.

Myth 12: You don't need a professional hairstylist anymore because you can just use YouTube videos

While YouTube instructional videos are fantastic resources, they can never give you the personal attention that a good professional hairstylist can give your hair (the key word being *good*). So continue to learn as much as you can from YouTube videos but don't ditch your hairstylist if they are good with your hair, knowledgeable and treat you right.

Myth 13: You should entrust all your hair care decisions to your hair stylist.

On the flip side of never going to see a hairstylist is having your hairstylist make all the decisions about your hair care. Far too many women have hair salon disaster stories because they blindly accepted what was suggested by a hairstylist. Become knowledgeable about your hair and next time you're in the salon, question anything that you are not sure of.

Myth 14: Black hair has a slower growth rate.

Another myth believed by far too many women. Black hair grows an average ½ an inch per month — the same average as Caucasian and Asian hair. This myth has probably spread due to our hair looking shorter when it is in its natural tightly coiled curl pattern.

Myth 15: Your natural hair is hard to maintain

This is a popular myth that is just not true. Natural hair is only hard to maintain if you are not sure how to maintain it. Once you learn how to take care of your natural hair and it becomes part of your routine it will be much easier than you might have thought.

CHAPTER TWO

TRANSITIONING TO NATURAL HAIR

What is transitioning ? Transitioning is the process of going from chemically relaxed hair to your natural hair. An ever growing number of black women are deciding to stop using relaxers and wear their hair natural. Being natural gives you a wider range of options when styling your hair and you avoid damage done by chemical relaxers.

Options you have when going natural

If you are considering going natural, there are several ways to transition:

1. Big Chop (BC)

A big chop is the act of cutting off all your relaxed hair in one sitting. You can do the big chop by yourself using shears/clippers and a mirror. However, when you do it yourself, you may end up with uneven hair especially in areas on the back of your head. If you decide to do it yourself make sure you use a clipper guard. A clipper guard is meant to leave a set amount of hair length. Alternatively (and the easier option), you can have a barber or hairstylist do it for you.

Pros of Big Chopping:

- You get rid of breaking and damaged hair in one sitting.
- As your hair grows out, you only have to deal with one texture.

Cons of Big Chopping:

- You may not be used to having very short hair, which for some women can be a very emotional experience.
- You will have limited styling options until your hair grows back.

2. Sew in Weave or Braids

The second option when it comes to transitioning is wearing

a weave or braiding your hair. You let your natural hair grow under the weave/braids and cut off your relaxed ends as your natural hair grows longer. Ideally, you should take out your weave or braids every 6 to 8 weeks to trim the hair.

Pros of Sew-in Weaves and Braids:

- Variety of styling options with weaves and braids as your natural hair gets to grow.
- You don't have to deal with two different textures of hair.

Cons of wearing Weaves and Braids:

- Your hair underneath may become neglected.
- Braids done too tight can cause hair loss.

3. Growing out your natural hair with your relaxed hair

The third option is growing out your natural hair with your relaxed hair. This is a way of transitioning already familiar to women who "stretch" their relaxer. If you are not familiar with stretching relaxer, just think of it as extending the time between relaxer touch ups. Growing out your natural hair can be done in as little as several weeks or it can go for months until you are satisfied with the length of your new growth. Once you are satisfied with your new growth, you can cut off the relaxed hair.

Pros to growing out your natural hair with your relaxed hair:

- A familiar process if you stretch your relaxer.
- You don't have to deal with short natural hair.

Cons to growing out your natural hair with your relaxed hair:

- Dealing with two textures can be difficult.
- You will get constant breakage at the line of demarcation (the point where your natural hair meets your relaxed hair).

So how do you know which is the best way for you to transition?

The Best Way To Transition

There is no single best way to transition. It's all about your goals, needs and wants. To best illustrate this, below is a map of two cities in a imaginary country called Hair. We will call the two cities—Relaxed City and Natural City.

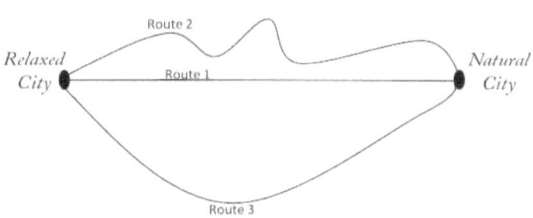

Figure 6. From Relaxed City to Natural City map

As you can see there are several ways to get to Natural City from Relaxed City. If someone were to ask you, "what is the best way to get to Natural City from Relaxed City?" — you would need more information. Do they prefer the shortest route with no scenery or do they prefer the longer route with scenic views ? The same applies to transitioning from relaxed hair to natural hair. It all depends on what you want whether you decide to big chop, transition with a weave or grow your natural hair out.

Is Natural Hair For You?

Use the following table as a guide to deciding   if going

natural is the right thing for you to do.

GO NATURAL IF:	DON'T GO NATURAL IF:
1. You are doing it for yourself, not to please someone else or be part of a trend.	1. You are completely happy with your relaxed or weave hair.
2. You have constant breakage and your hair is thinning due to chemically processing your hair.	2. You haven't done the research on how to take care of natural hair.
3. You want to save money on weaves and stylist visits.	3. You just don't have the patience or time to deal with your natural hair right now.
4. You want to have the healthiest hair possible.	4. You are only doing it because your best friend or favorite celebrity decided to go natural.
5. You want to have the many styling options that natural hair can give you at low to no cost.	5. You saw a couple of videos of natural hair tutorials on YouTube and you think it's cute and you want to try it out.
6. You want to participate in sports or swimming without having to worry too much about your hair.	6. You have been chastised by other women or men because you relax your hair or wear weave.

Keys to a successful transition

Transitioning to natural hair can be challenging and at times frustrating. Below are 13 tips to help and ease the transitioning process for you:

1. Patience

You will need patience with yourself as you learn to take care of your natural hair. You are going down a path that is new and unfamiliar to you. As black women, a great number of us have been relaxed since we were teenagers and it is important to realize that learning new hair care practices won't happen overnight.

You also need to be patient with your hair as you handle it. Be gentle with your hair when you are combing or brushing to avoid damage and breakage.

2. Doubt and Second Guessing Yourself

As you transition from relaxed to natural hair, it is important to realize that doubt and second guessing yourself on your decision to go natural is normal. There will be times when you get so frustrated with your hair, you will want to run to the store and buy a relaxer kit. There will be times when you look in the mirror and get emotional because you have really short hair. To have a successful transition, you have to realize that change is never easy and there will be challenges. All this is normal and part of the transitioning process.

3. Have "go to" hairstyles

Once you have done the big chop it is important to have certain "go-to" hair styles that are easy for you to do. When you plan ahead on which hairstyles you will wear, you will save yourself a lot of frustration.

So before you do the big chop, know if you will be wearing a wig or twists or locs until your hair is longer and you have more styling options. You don't want to be in a situation where you have done the big chop and you have no clue which hairstyle to wear.

4. Be ready to deal with Naysayers

When you go natural, there are some people that may not like it or criticize your decision. It's easy to brush off the random stranger on the street but what do you do with close friends, family or a spouse? Here are a few tips:

- First, hear them out and find out why they are against you going natural.
- Let them know you appreciate their concern but going natural is something you are doing for the health of your hair (or whichever reason you went natural). Educate them on the benefits of going natural.
- Ask for their support but if they are still not willing to support you, you will have to have the mental strength to continue being natural without their support. You will find tons of support on natural hair forums online.

5. Do you research

To have a successful transition, you will need to do your research and learn how to maintain natural hair before going natural. Take time to find out how to take care of your natural hair. Use all the resources available to you. Use this book, ask friends who are natural, use YouTube, use online forums — anything that's available to you.

6. Maintain your hair properly

Once you have done your research on how to take care of natural hair, you should apply what you learn. There is no point in just learning and not applying what you learn. Proper maintenance of your natural hair means detangling, washing, conditioning and moisturizing it. **Properly maintaining your natural hair is crucial to a successful transition**.

7. Keep focused on your goal

For most women who transition to natural hair, their goal is to have healthy hair. When transitioning you must always remember your goal and your initial motivation for going natural. Healthy hair doesn't happen overnight. If you've had years and years of bad hair care practices don't expect to have healthy hair overnight. It will take time and effort on your part. Keep focused on your goal.

8. Be okay with the unexpected

To have a successful transition, you must be okay with the unexpected. A frequent frustration of women who transition is an unexpected hair texture and a slower than expected hair growth rate. Some women before doing the big chop, expect their natural hair to be wavier or have a looser curl and are disappointed when they see that's not the case. Other women expect their hair will grow back fast and become frustrated at the slow pace of their hair growth.

To eliminate this frustration, before doing the Big Chop, say to yourself "I will be ok with my natural hair texture and the speed at which it grows."

9. Avoid Heat

Once you have decided to go natural, try your best to avoid direct heat on your hair. Excessive heat is damaging to the hair and if you continue practices that are damaging to your hair, you will end up with the same problems you wanted to avoid in the first place.

If you must use heat make sure you always use a heat protectant and use low to medium heat settings.

10. Say "NO" to Texturizer

Just like heat, you want to avoid using texturizer on your hair. The temptation is greatest when your hair is short and you have limited styling options or when you are not happy with your natural curl pattern. *Don't do it*. This will just set you back on your transition. Texturizers work the same way relaxers do. Make a promise to yourself that you won't use a texturizer once you have made the decision to go natural.

11. Accessorize

A common complaint among women who fear doing the big chop and having short hair is that they won't look "feminine enough". Having short hair is a great time to use accessories to accentuate your look. It's a time to experiment with hair accessories and earrings. Try out hoop earrings, flowers, decorative clips and stylish head bands. Have fun with your short hair as you transition!

12. Find inspiration and motivation

Having inspiration and motivation is key to a successful transition. You can find both from natural hair forums online. Most forum members are more than willing to help newly naturals navigate their natural hair journey.

Facebook groups and YouTube are also a great place to see pictures of women who have beautiful natural hairstyles. Whenever you feel like giving up on your natural hair journey look for motivation and inspiration in online communities.

13. Find a professional natural hairstylist

If you are not comfortable or don't think you have done enough research on maintaining your natural hair, seek out a professional natural hairstylist. Having a good natural hairstylist can be the difference between successfully transitioning or going back to relaxing your hair. When you are looking for a natural hairstylist, make sure they specialize in natural hair and are well reviewed.

If you live in a small city, it can be difficult to find a natural hairstylist and it may mean looking for one in the nearest large city.

CHAPTER THREE

MAINTAINING AND PROTECTING YOUR NATURAL HAIR

Having healthy, beautiful hair is something that doesn't happen by accident. It will require effort on your part. Our hair needs to be maintained and protected to remain healthy. To do this, you will need to have a hair care regimen and *follow it*. A hair care regimen can be complicated with lots of steps or it can be simple with just a few steps. This chapter will go over the six steps you should include in your own regimen to have healthy, beautiful hair. The six steps to maintaining healthy, beautiful hair are:

1. Detangling
2. Washing
3. Conditioning

Six steps to healthy, beautiful hair

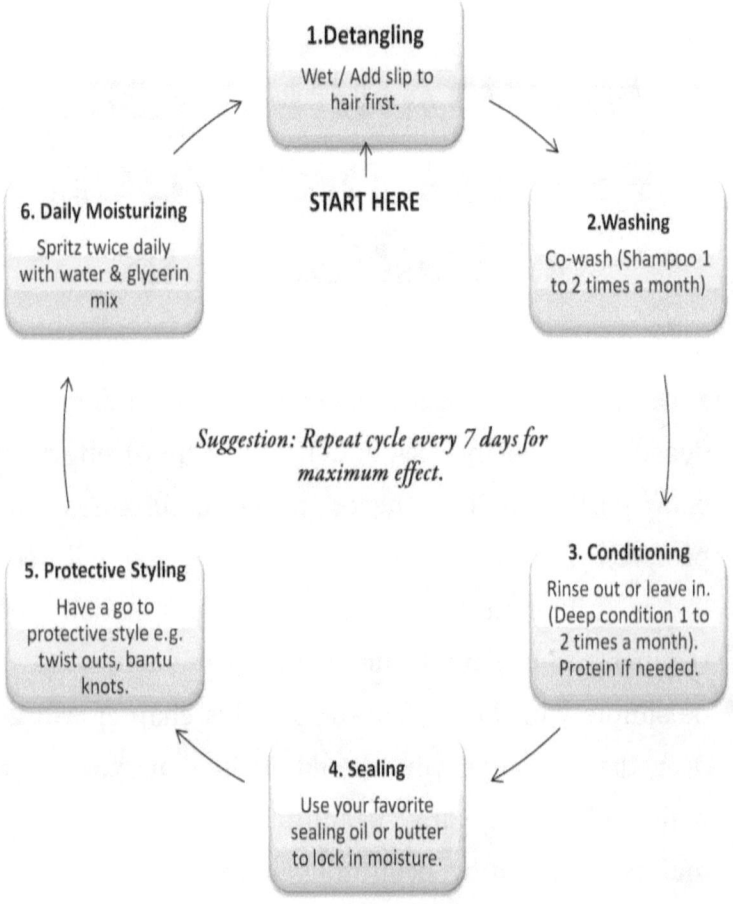

Figure 6. Illustration showing the necessary steps in a hair care regimen

4. Sealing

5. Protective Styling

6. Daily Moisturizing

Will discuss them one at a time starting with detangling.

1. Detangling

What causes knots and tangles in the first place? The unique nature of our hair means that it knots and tangles more often than straight Caucasian and Asian hair. Why is that? Our hair curls which makes it easier for hair strands to intertwine and knot together. Another way to understand knots and tangles, is to think of all the power and video cables behind your TV stand. It almost seems as if they tangle and knot up without any extra help from anyone. It's the same with your hair.

Another reason our hair gets tangled up is shedding hair. Shedding hair is hair that has reached the end of its normal growth cycle and falls off. Instead of the shed hair falling to the ground, it gets intertwined with other hair strands and does not fall to the ground. Regular washing of your hair limits knots and tangles due to shedding hair.

Detangling should always be done first. Detangling is first on the list because without detangling first — everything else that follows might actually do more harm than good to your hair! Hair with knots and tangles is more likely to break when you are handling it through washing, conditioning or styling.

Since your hair is best detangled when moist, detangling can be done in the shower or over the sink. It's up to you. Before you start detangling, either spray a water and glycerin mixture or apply a conditioner to your hair. You are making the hair soft so it can be ready for detangling. This process is called *plasticizing* the hair.

Finger Detangling and Wide tooth comb detangling. After you're done plasticizing your hair, gently run your fingers through the hair, detangling any large knots and tangles. This step requires you to have extra patience as it can be easy to use too much force which may lead to unnecessary breakage.

After finger detangling, follow up with a wide

tooth comb to get rid of any knots that you missed while finger detangling. So, to summarize detangling:

1. Only detangle moist/plasticized hair.
2. Finger detangle first.
3. Follow up with a wide tooth comb.

After you are done detangling, the next step is washing your hair.

2. Washing

The second step in the healthy, beautiful hair regimen is washing. Washing your hair is done to remove dirt, shed hair, sweat and product build up. Whenever you go for long periods of time without washing your hair, you risk dirt and product build up which will eventually clog up your pores and cause excessive dandruff.

Options when washing your hair

When it comes to washing your hair , you can either use a conditioner (called *co-washing*) or you can use a shampoo. The reason you would want to avoid using a shampoo is because most shampoos have an extremely drying effect on your hair and with our hair already naturally dry , excessive use of shampoo leads to increased breakage.

Will go over co-washing and shampooing:

1. *Co-Washing*

Co-washing is short for conditioner washing. It is an excellent alternative to shampooing your hair. Co-washing uses conditioner as a replacement for shampoo. A benefit of co-washing is that it's not as drying as shampoo and does not strip your hair of its natural oil.   Another benefit of co-washing is that it can be done more frequently than shampooing. Co-washing is ideal for women who exercise daily to remove sweat build up without the drying effects of shampoo.

How to Co-Wash

Step 1:

Choose a moisturizing conditioner. Preferably an inexpensive one, as you will be using lots of it.

Step 2:

Section your hair into 4 or more sections.

Step 3:

Wet your hair with luke warm water. Apply the conditioner generously to your scalp and hair from root to tip.

Step 4:

Rub scalp with the pads of your fingers removing dirt and product build up.

Step 5:

Rinse out with luke warm or cold water.

2. *Shampooing*

As good as co-washing is, it alone is not enough to remove build up of product that happens over time. Silicones in conditioners also add to product build up. Alternating between co-washing and shampooing your hair becomes necessary to remove product build up .

When shampooing, you should concentrate on the scalp. Using the pads (bottom) of your fingers gently rub in the shampoo, agitating the dirt and product build up. Never use your finger nails as your scalp can become scratched, leaving it vulnerable to bacterial infections.

Different types of shampoo

All shampoos can be placed in one of two categories - cleansers or combo cleanser conditioners.

1. **Cleansers** : Cleansers are shampoos that contain ingredients that cleanse the hair. Because cleansers strip the hair of its natural oil, they must always be followed up with a conditioner.

2. **Combo cleanser and conditioner (2-in-1)** : Combo cleanser and conditioners are shampoos that contain ingredients that cleanse the hair as well as condition it. These 2-in-1 shampoos do not do as good a job when compared to using a shampoo and a separate conditioner

Different marketing terms for shampoos

You will find different terms used by companies to describe the shampoos they sell:

i) Hydrating or Moisturizing shampoo
ii) Clarifying shampoo
iii) Chelating shampoo
iv) Anti-dandruff shampoo

Here is a guide to understanding what this all means.

i) *Hydrating or Moisturizing shampoo* : Is a shampoo formulated to add moisture to the hair. It does this by having one or more humectants. Humectants are substances that absorb moisture from the air. Common humectants are glycerine, propylene glycol and panthenol.

ii) **Clarifying shampoo** : Is a shampoo that is formulated to remove product build up, chlorine and mineral deposits. Clarifying shampoo is also good for swimmers to remove chlorine build up.

iii) **Chelating shampoo** : A chelating shampoo is similar to a clarifying shampoo, however it is formulated to remove mineral deposits. Chelating shampoo is good for those who live in hard water areas and to remove mineral deposits when you use a no lye relaxer.

iv) **Anti-dandruff shampoo** : An anti-dandruff shampoo is a shampoo that is formulated to remove and prevent dandruff. Anti-dandruff shampoos do not all have the same active ingredient. Common active ingredients are *selenium sulfide, zinc pyrithione, coal tar, ketoconazole* and *salicylic acid*. If you find that one anti-dandruff shampoo is not working for you, you can try one with a different active ingredient.

Do you have hard water?

Hard water is water that has a high content of minerals. When you wash your hair with hard water, minerals such as lime and calcium are deposited. These minerals build up and will dry your hair causing breakage.

If you live in a known hard water state (Arizona, Kansas, New Mexico, Texas and parts of Southern California) you will want to include a chelating shampoo as part of your regimen or purchase a shower head filter.

Deciding which shampoo to use

With so many options when it comes to shampoos, how do you know which one is the best for your hair? Some things to consider when picking a shampoo:

1. *Using a gentle or harsh shampoo*

Most shampoos contain sulfates. Sulfates are substances that leave your hair and scalp clean, but in the process strip your hair of its natural oils and may irritate your scalp. This can lead to dry, brittle hair which is susceptible to breakage and also excessive dandruff due to an irritated scalp. Two sulfates that are considered "harsh" are *Sodium Lauryl Sulfate* (SLS) and *Sodium Lauryl Ether Sulfate* (SLES).

Gentle shampoos are shampoos that are sulfate free or contain a "mild" sulfate. While gentle shampoos are great because they don't strip the oil off your hair, some may not be as cleansing if you happen to have a lot of product build up. The trick is finding a shampoo that is effective but not harsh on your hair.

2. *What is the pH of the shampoo?*

When picking a shampoo you want one that is as close to the natural pH of your hair (4.5 to 5.5) as possible. Unless you have low porosity hair, regular use of a shampoo with an alkaline pH (above 7) is not recommend and can be damaging to your hair.

3. *Swimming and hard water*

If you swim you will need to use a clarifying shampoo

to remove chlorine build up. If you live in a hard water area, you will want to include a chelating shampoo as part of your regimen.

4. Do you have excessive dandruff?

If you have excessive dandruff, you want to include an anti-dandruff shampoo in your regimen. An anti-dandruff shampoo **should not** be used as a permanent solution to dandruff. Find out what the underlying cause of your excessive dandruff is.

3. Conditioning

The third step in the healthy, beautiful hair regimen is conditioning. Conditioning is done to improve the "condition" of your hair by restoring moisture and strength. Hair can easily be damaged by the weather, heat, chemicals and excessive brushing. Frequent use of a conditioner is needed because the effects of a conditioner are not permanent. There are 2 types of conditioner:

The 2 types of conditioners

All conditioners can be placed in one of two categories — either *leave-in* or *rinse out* conditioner.

Leave-in conditioner : Leave-in conditioners are made with ingredients that are meant to be left on the hair and at the same time not weigh your hair down. Leave-in conditioners, in general, are thinner than rinse out conditioners and are usually found as sprays or light creams.

Rinse out conditioner : Rinse out conditioners are made with ingredients that are meant to 'stick' to your hair and continue to work even after rinsing. Rinse out conditioners are thicker and heavier than leave-in conditioners. A rinse out conditioner will weigh your hair down if not rinsed out.

Different terms used for conditioner

You will find different terms used by companies to describe the conditioners they sell:

i) Deep conditioner

ii) Moisturizing conditioner

iii) Protein conditioner

iv) Heat protectant

v) Detangling conditioner

Below is description of what this all means:

i) **Deep conditioner** : Is a rinse out conditioner that is usually meant to be left on the hair for about 30 minutes or more and then rinsed out. Heat is often used with a deep conditioner to increase effectiveness.

ii) **Moisturizing Conditioner** : Is a rinse out or leave in conditioner that's formulated to restore moisture to your hair. Water should be the first ingredient in a moisturizing conditioner. Moisturizing conditioners contain humectants which help in the absorption of moisture. Since our hair is naturally dry, moisturizing conditioners are an absolute necessity in Black hair care.

iii) **Protein conditioner** : Is a rinse out or leave-in conditioner that's formulated to restore strength to your hair. Protein conditioners are generally recommended for hair that has been damaged by heat or chemicals. Some women may find they are allergic to the protein in protein conditioners and may want to skip them all together.

iv) **Heat protectant** : Is a leave-in conditioner that is formulated to slow down the transfer of heat and protect the hair from heat damage.

v) **Detangling conditioner** : Is a rinse-out conditioner that is formulated to assist in detangling of the hair. Detangling conditioners often contain silicones which smooth the hair, making it easier for a comb or fingers to go through the hair.

4. Sealing

Sealing is the fourth step in the healthy, beautiful hair regimen. After you have used a leave in conditioner or moisturizer of your choice, sealing is the process of locking in that moisture. Without sealing the moisture, your hair is more likely to dry out sooner.

Oils and butters are used to seal in moisture.

Oils and butters are good for sealing in moisture because the water molecules are too big to pass through the oil or butter. While oils and butters are effective at locking in the moisture — the process of sealing is not permanent. The oil or butter must be reapplied every time you condition your hair. So how do you decide which oil or butter to use? Will go over the different types of oils and butters.

Which oils to use

Penetrating vs. Coating oils. All oils are not created the same. Oils differ in what they can do and when it comes to sealing in moisture, oils can be divided into two groups — penetrating oils and coating oils.

Penetrating oils are oils that are able to penetrate the cuticle and get into the cortex. Penetrating oils are best used as a pre-shampoo (pre-poo) treatment or mixed into your conditioner as a leave-in conditioner. Examples of penetrating oils are: *coconut oil, olive oil and avocado oil.*

Coating oils are oils that are not able to penetrate the cuticle. They coat the cuticle forming a layer that prevents moisture from escaping. Examples of coating oils are : *Jamaican Black Castor Oil, Grape seed oil, Jojoba Oil.* These oils are good to use for sealing in moisture.

Food grade vs. Cosmetic grade oils. When purchasing penetrating or coating oils, always make sure you are purchasing food grade oils. To make sure you are purchasing food grade oils, go to the cooking oil section of your grocery store. Food grade oils are often marked as Cold Pressed or Extra Virgin. Food grade oils are purer than the cosmetic grade oils and still have most of their nutrients — making them the best option for your hair.

Let's now look at the butters.

Which butters to use

Just like oils, butters can be used for sealing in moisture. Butters tend to work best for those with thicker hair or high porosity hair. Examples of sealing butters are : *Shea butter, Mango butter.*

5. Protective Styling

The fifth step in the healthy, beautiful hair care regimen is protective styling. A protective style is a hair style that protects your hair from breakage by either tucking the ends away or lifting them off your shoulders and clothing.

Protective styles are a great way to protect your hair in the summer and winter months from extreme weather. There are dozens of protective styles that you can choose from. When protective styling, you can do a simple bun or if you have more time you can do twists, it will come down to how much time you have and your personal preference.

6. Daily Moisturizing

The sixth step of the healthy, beautiful hair regimen is daily moisturizing. Even after sealing in the moisture on wash day, your hair still needs daily moisture. Over time your hair loses the sealed in moisture through evaporation. So how do you moisturize daily?

A good daily moisturizing technique is to spray your

hair with a few short bursts of a water and glycerin mix (do it at least twice a day). This is called *spritzing*. Water is an ideal moisturizer and glycerin is a humectant — meaning it absorbs moisture from the air.

For your water and glycerin mix, you will need to mix in one part glycerin ($1/5$) for every four parts of water ($4/5$) into a spray bottle. If you find your mix to be too sticky, add some more water to dilute. You can also add essential oils for fragrance.

Winter Warning: Some women find the water and glycerin mix drying for their hair during the winter months. If you find this is the case for you, you can use a water and Aloe Vera juice mix. Mix in one part Aloe Vera ($1/3$) for every two parts of Water ($2/3$).

When spritzing make sure to spray the ends of your hair. The ends of your hair are the oldest as well as the driest part of your hair. They need all the moisture they can get.

Tips to creating your own regimen

1. *Set aside a specific day and keep to it*. Setting aside a specific day out of the week as your wash day creates a routine and eventually it becomes habit. Your wash day should be a day when you have enough time to do your hair without being in a rush. Having an irregular wash day can lead to product build up, dry hair and breakage.

2. *Don't rush*. Once you have selected a specific day out the week, it is important not to be in a rush when doing your hair. Being in a rush can cause rough handling which can lead to breakage. Take your time and be gentle with your hair.

3. *Don't overcomplicate*. Don't over complicate your regimen. A mistake that some women make is to over complicate their regimen, which leads to frustration and you end up dreading wash day. Washing your hair should not be an all day event that stops you from doing other things. When you have an overcomplicated regimen you may end up neglecting your hair because you keep procrastinating your wash day.

Simplify your regimen, have it fit into your life rather than making your life fit into your regimen and you will look forward to your wash days.

4. *Pick products and accessories that are good for your hair.* Be mindful of the products and accessories you use, making sure you are reading ingredient labels to see what's in the product.

You should also make sure the hair accessories you're using are not damaging to your hair. Common accessories like rubber bands and fine tooth combs can be damaging to your hair.

Protecting your hair while you sleep

To prevent matting and breakage, it is essential to protect your hair when you go to sleep each night. When sleeping on a cotton pillow case, the constant rubbing and friction of your hair against the cotton fabric can cause knots and tangles which leads to breakage. Follow these tips to protect your hair while sleeping:

1. *Wrap up your hair.* To protect your hair while you

sleep, you will need to wrap a silk/satin scarf around your hair. Silk and satin are much smoother than cotton and will cause less friction on your hair.

2. *Silk pillowcase.* While wrapping up your hair with a silk/satin scarf is good, some women find that the scarf will come loose or fall off while they are sleeping. If this were to happen, for added protection to your hair, get a silk/satin pillow case.

Protecting your hair while you exercise

When exercising you want to protect your hair from salt build up. Sweat left on the hair will cause a buildup of salt. The salt will dry your hair and eventually lead to breakage. To prevent this from happening to you, use these tips when working out:

1. *Wear a sweat headband.* A sweat headband will absorb most of the sweat when you exercise.

2. *High pony tail or bun.* Wear your hair up in a ponytail or bun to prevent sweat getting to it.

3. *Co-wash or gentle shampoo*. The sweat headband should absorb most of the sweat. You can get away with not washing your hair after a light workout. However, after a heavy work out or several light workouts you want to co-wash or use a gentle shampoo to wash your hair.

Protecting your hair while you swim

When you go swimming you want to protect your hair from chlorine damage. To protect your hair while swimming use these tips:

1. *Apply a protective barrier*. Before going in the pool either soak your hair with fresh tap water or apply coconut oil from the roots to the tips of your hair. This acts as a protective barrier to prevent chlorine from getting absorbed into your hair.

2. *Swim cap*. Put on a swim cap as an extra layer of protection against the chlorine.

3. *Rinse hair*. Once you are done swimming, rinse your hair with fresh tap water.

4. *Shampoo and Condition*. Use a clarifying shampoo to remove the chlorine and follow up with a conditioner.

MAINTAINING AND PROTECTING YOUR NATURAL HAIR

CHAPTER FOUR

SELECTING YOUR PRODUCTS

When it comes to products you have hundreds of options to choose from. You have the inexpensive or the expensive, the natural or the organic, the ones labeled for Black hair and the ones that don't say for Black hair. With all these options, it can easily get confusing. How then do you know which products are best for your hair ? These tips will help you out:

1. *Your hair can't tell the difference between an expensive product and an inexpensive one.* Your hair only knows if a product is good for it or bad for it, not how much you paid for it. When deciding which conditioner or shampoo to use, always look at the ingredients to see what's in the product. Ask yourself, why does it cost so much? You will find that products with similar ingredients can have a big price

difference and you are just paying for the brand name.

2. *When buying a product for the first time, get a sample or buy the smallest size available.* Often you buy a shampoo or conditioner based on a recommendation but just because it worked for the person that recommended it to you doesn't mean it will work the same for you as well. Save your money and buy the smallest size first — and if it works then you can go back and buy a bigger size.

3. *Spot test new products.* When you get a new product or new oil, place a very small amount (about a dime size) on the inside of your elbow for at least 24 hours and then wash it off. If you experience swelling or burning then stop using the product or oil.

4. *For discounts follow your favorite product manufacturer on Facebook and Twitter.* Often companies will post exclusive sales and coupon codes on social media.

5. *In general, products with the fewest ingredients are usually the best for your hair.* When a product has dozens of ingredients listed on the bottle, it increases the chance of an allergic reaction.

6. *Look for products with ingredients you can pronounce.* If you are having a difficult time pronouncing an ingredient on the bottle, do your research and find out what that ingredient is and what it does for your hair.

7. *You can use products that are marketed to white women or women of other races.* Just because a product doesn't say on the box its meant for Black hair doesn't mean it's not good for your hair. Just make sure you are checking the ingredient list not just picking a product because it says it's for "Black hair".

8. *Use Amazon's Subscribe and Save program to save money when buying shampoos, conditioners or any other hair product.* Amazon.com has a great selection of shampoos, conditioners, oils and butters. Use their Subscribe and Save program and you can save up to 15%.

9. *Try out product box subscription services.* For a monthly fee (usually ranging between $10 to $30) you can receive a package that contains several products every month. This allows you to try out new products and also save on paying full retail price on products.

10. *Avoid the urge to become a product junkie.* Sometimes as women we try and find that one product that will solve all our hair problems. We end up spending lots of money on products that may actually be damaging to our hair. Avoid this temptation and you will save yourself a lot of money.

Recommended products for your regimen

Recommended commercial moisturizing conditioners

Herbal Essences Hello Hydration
Nexxus Humectress Ultimate Moisturizing
Tresemme Naturals Nourishing Moisture

Recommended commercial protein conditioners

ORS Repleneshing Pak
Aubrey Organics GPB
Joico K-Pak Reconstruct

Recommended commercial detangling conditioners

Aussie Moist Conditioner
Mane 'n Tail Detangler

Recommended commercial shampoos

L'Oreal Evercreme Intense Nourishing shampoo
Trader Joes Tea Tingle shampoo
Aubrey Organics Green Tea Clarifying shampoo

Recommended sealing oils and butters

Jojoba oil
Jamaican Black Castor Oil
Grape seed oil
Coconut oil
Olive oil
Shea Butter
Mango butter
Cocoa Butter

Recommended styling creams and gels

One 'n Only Argan Oil Styling Cream

Shea Moisture Coconut & Hibiscus Curling Soufflé

Shea Moisture Coconut & Hibiscus Curl Enhancing
Smoothie

Eco Styler Olive Oil Styling Gel

Curls Curl Crème Brule

CHAPTER FIVE

ADVANCED HAIR CARE METHODS

While usually not part of a regular hair care regimen, advanced hair care methods when used at the appropriate time will do your hair a world of good.

The advanced hair care methods will go over are:

1. Protein treatments.
2. Hot oil treatments.
3. L.O.C, L.C.O and L.C.S.O.
4. Hair steaming.
5. Pre-poo treatments.
6. Scalp massages.
7. Baggying.

1. Protein treatments

What is it?

A protein treatment (also referred to as a re-constructor) is a hair conditioning treatment done to add protein to your hair. Since your hair is largely made up of protein, a protein treatment will add strength and repair damaged hair.

When to do a protein treatment?

Protein treatments should only be done to hair that has been damaged due to heat, coloring or relaxing. Using a protein treatment when your hair does not need one can lead to major hair breakage. Be careful when deciding when to use a protein treatment.

Even when your hair does need a protein treatment — protein treatments should be limited to no more than once every 6 weeks. Doing a protein treatment more than once every 6 weeks can be very damaging to your hair.

Examples of Protein Treatments: *Aphoghee Two-step treatment protein for damaged hair, Mizani Kerafuse intense strengthening treatment.*

What it does?

Strengthens and repairs hair damaged by chemical processing, coloring and heat.

2. Hot oil treatments

What is it?

A hot oil treatment is a hair conditioning treatment done to condition and repair damaged hair using oil and heat.

How to do a hot oil treatment

Step 1:

Pour a ¼ cup of your favorite oil (or you can use a mix of oils) into a bowl.

Step 2:

Dip your fingers into the bowl. Using the pads of your fingers, massage the oil onto your scalp. Apply remaining oil onto your hair, making sure to apply from the roots to the ends.

Step 3:

Cover your hair with a plastic cap and sit under a hooded dryer for 15 minutes. (With no hooded dryer, you can wrap a warm towel over the plastic cap and let it sit for 30 minutes).

Step 4:

Co - wash your hair to rinse out the oil. Apply your leave-in conditioner.

Which oils to use

Good oils to use for a hot oil treatment are avocado oil, olive oil, coconut oil and jojoba oil. When doing a hot oil treatment for the first time, make sure not to use more than one oil. The reason you want to use only one oil at first is because you may be allergic to certain oils and if you use multiple oils at once, you won't know which oil you are allergic to.

How often?

Hot oil treatments can be done once a month.

3. L.O.C, L.C.O, L.C.S.O

L.O.C, L.C.O and L.C.S.O are acronyms for methods used to moisturize constantly dry hair. The letters in each acronym are in sequential order of applying the product to your hair. These methods work well because they add extra layers to seal in moisture, reducing the rate that moisture evaporates from your hair.

Deciding which method works best for your hair comes down to personal preference. If you find your hair to be constantly dry, you may want to try each one of these methods and eventually settle on the method that works best for you.

The L.O.C Method

Step 1: (L) for Liquid:

To damp hair, apply a water based leave-in conditioner or spritz your hair with water.

Step 2: (O) for Oil:

Apply an oil of your choice to seal in the moisture.

Step 3: (C) for Cream:

Once you have sealed in the moisture with an oil of your choice, apply a cream (butter) to your hair to add an extra layer to seal in the moisture. An example of a good butter is Shea butter.

The L.C.O Method

Step 1: (L) for Liquid:

To damp hair, Apply a water based leave-in conditioner or spritz your hair with water.

Step 2: (C) for Cream:

Apply a cream (butter) e.g. Shea butter as the first layer for sealing in the moisture.

Step 3: (O) for Oil:

Apply an oil of your choice as the second layer to seal in the moisture.

The L.C.S.O Method

Step 1: (L) for Liquid:

To damp hair, apply a water based leave-in conditioner or spritz your hair with water.

Step 2: (C) for Cream:

Apply a cream (butter) as the first layer for sealing in the moisture.

Step 3: (S) for Styler:

Apply a setting lotion as the second layer to seal in the moisture.

Step 4: (O) for Oil:

Apply an oil of your choice as the third layer to seal in the moisture.

4. Hair steaming

What is it?

Hair steaming is a method of conditioning and moisturizing your hair. The benefits to steaming your hair are:

1. *It increases the blood circulation in your scalp for improved hair growth.*

2. *Moisturizes your hair.* Your hair needs moisture to remain healthy and prevent dryness.

3. *Cleanses the scalp of product buildup and dirt.* Clogged pores on your scalp prevent hair growth.

4. *Reduces dandruff.* By cleaning the scalp, the dead skin cells are removed.

How do you steam your hair?

Get a personal hair steamer. These can be purchased from a

variety of websites online. A good personal hair steamer is the Huetiful hair steamer and can be purchased at www.behuetiful.com.

5. Pre-Poo treatments

What is it?

Pre-poo is short for pre-shampoo. It is a hair conditioning treatment done to protect your hair from the ingredients found in shampoos. These ingredients called *sulfates* clean your hair but also strip your hair of its natural oils.

How to Pre-poo

Step 1:

Pick an oil of your choice. A good oil to use is olive oil. You can also use avocado oil or coconut oil.

Step 2:

Section off your hair into 4 or more manageable sections. Apply the oil generously to each section (you can use a spray bottle for easier application).

Step 3:

Place a plastic shower cap over your hair and let it sit. After 30 to 35 minutes remove the shower cap (alternatively you can sit under a hooded dryer for 15 to 20 minutes)

Step 4:

You can now detangle and shampoo your hair as normal.

When to do it?

A pre-poo treatment should be done before you shampoo your hair.

6. Scalp Massages

What is it

A scalp massage is a great way to relieve tension and stimulate the hair follicles by improving blood circulation. Scalp massages are an excellent hair growth aid.

How to do it

There are two ways to do a scalp massage 1) using your hands only and 2) using oil.

1) *Using your hands only*

Step 1:

Using the pads of your fingers gently massage your forehead for about 30 seconds.

Step 2:

Parting your hair, start massaging your scalp in circular motions working your way to the nape. Make sure you cover the entire scalp.

Step 3:

Once you reach the nape, continue massaging in circular motions working your way back to the forehead.

The entire scalp massage should take you between 5 to 10 minutes.

2) Using oil

Step 1:

Place a small amount of your favorite oil into a bowl. Dip the pads of your fingers into the bowl.

Step 2:

Beginning at your forehead, start massaging your scalp in circular motions until you get to the nape.

Step 3:

Dip the pads of your fingers in the oil again and continue massaging, working your way back to your forehead.

When to do it

You can do a scalp massage daily before going to sleep or once a week on wash day.

7. Baggying

What is it

Baggying or the Baggy method is a great way to moisturize dry hair by using a moisturizer, an oil and a plastic cap or bag.

How to do it

Step 1:

Apply a water based leave-in conditioner or spritz your hair with water.

Step 2:

Seal in the moisture with an oil of your choice.

Step 3:

Cover your hair with a plastic cap or bag.

Step 4:

Leave the plastic cap on for 30 minutes and then remove (some women choose to leave it on overnight).

When to do it

Once a week after you have washed your hair or any other day before you go to sleep.

CHAPTER SIX

BAD HAIR CARE HABITS

Are you guilty of one of these bad hair care habits? Unfortunately, the habits below are far too common. Avoid them to get healthy, beautiful hair.

1. *Combing your hair from the roots.* When you comb your hair starting at the roots you increase the likelihood of snagging and breakage. Also, combing from the roots can be painful because you are pulling your hair so close to the nerve endings. Always start combing at the ends of your hair and work your way up.

2. *Being impatient and rushing when using a fine tooth comb.* This is a common practice that is bad for your hair. Rushing and being impatient when using a fine tooth comb will lead to hair snagging and breakage. Whenever you use a fine tooth comb on your hair take extra care to be gentle.

3. *Using hot water to wash your hair.* Hot water can be very drying to our already dry hair. Stick to washing your hair with luke warm water and for a final rinse use cold water. Cold water closes the cuticles, helps to lock in the moisture and increases the shine of your hair.

4. *Towel drying your hair.* Drying hair by rubbing it with a towel is a fairly common bad hair care practice. The rubbing motion causes friction which leads to damage and breakage. A much better way to dry your hair is to wrap it up in an old cotton T-shirt for about 5 minutes. The t-shirt will absorb most of the water without the damage that a towel does.

5. *Blow drying dripping wet hair.* Blow drying dripping wet hair is damaging to your hair. Before using a blow dryer, wrap your hair in an old T-shirt for 5 minutes and let it air dry for another 5 minutes. Apply a heat protectant and use the blow dryer only on a low to medium heat setting.

6. *Completely drying your hair with a blow dryer.* Drying you hair a 100% when using a blow dryer is damaging to your hair. You want to make sure you do not completely dry it out. Leave a little moisture in your hair and let it air dry.

7. *Multiple passes when flat ironing.* Multiple passes over the same section of hair can be very damaging. You don't want to burn your hair. Limit your passes to one or two at most.

BAD HAIR CARE HABITS

CHAPTER SEVEN

GOOD HAIR CARE HABITS

1. *Moisturizing your hair.* Our hair is dry and keeping it moisturized is good hair care. From a moisturizing conditioner on wash day to a daily moisturizer, your hair will appreciate it and you will reduce breakage caused by dry hair.

2. *Protective styling.* While it is tempting to wear your hair out, wearing it in a protective style protects the ends and helps you to retain length.

3. *Sealing in moisture.* Whenever you apply your leave in conditioner or moisturizer it is important to seal the moisture in. Sealing in the moisture keeps your hair moisturized by slowing down the loss of moisture through

evaporation.

4. *Deep conditioning.* Deep conditioning is a very effective way to restore your hair's condition, providing it with both moisture and strength. Deep condition at least 1 to 2 times a month to keep your hair nourished and reduce damage.

5. *Low manipulation.* Avoid constant brushing, combing and styling of your hair. This reduces the likelihood of breakage and damage when handling your hair.

6. *Using a heat protectant.* Whenever you apply heat to your hair make sure you apply a heat protectant first. A heat protectant prevents damage to your hair by slowing down the transfer of heat.

7. *Finger detangling.* Before using a comb to detangle, finger detangle first. Finger detangling allows you to be more gentle with your hair and you don't have to worry about breakage from a comb getting snagged in a knot.

8. *Cutting off your split ends.* The sooner you cut off your split ends the better it is for your hair. Neglecting to cut off

split ends will allow the split to travel further up the hair shaft leading to more damage and breakage.

CHAPTER EIGHT

GROWING YOUR HAIR LONG

The two biggest myths when it comes to Black women and growing long hair is that Black women can't grow long hair and "you have to be mixed" to have long hair. Nothing could be further from the truth. Unfortunately, these myths have been repeated so many times that many black women now believe it's the truth.

The truth is that Black women can grow long hair and the secret is **retaining length**. As Black women, we have a unique challenge in retaining length because our hair is naturally dry and prone to breakage. This chapter will give you all the information you need to retain length and grow your hair longer.

Understanding Hair Growth

Understanding how your hair grows is a good starting point to growing your hair long. Hair growth happens in 3 stages - Anagen, Catagen and Telogen.

The Hair Growth Cycle

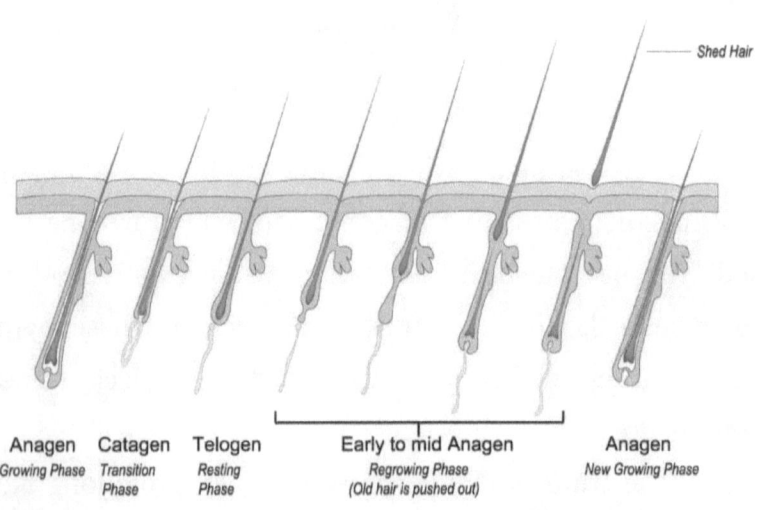

Figure 8. Illustration of the Hair Growth Cycle

The Phases of Hair Growth

Anagen

Anagen is the growing phase of the hair. The anagen phase

can last from between 2 to 6 years and <u>the longer your hair stays in the anagen phase the longer it will grow</u>. On average hair grows ½ an inch every month while in the anagen phase. At any one time around 85% of your hair is in the anagen phase.

Catagen

The catagen phase is a transition phase and is the shortest period lasting between 1 to 2 weeks. During the catagen phase, the supply of nutrients is cut off to the hair strand and your hair stops growing. At any one time, around 3% of your hair is in the catagen phase.

Telogen

The telogen phase is the resting phase and will last between 1 to 4 months. During this phase your hair follicle is at rest. Once the telogen phase is complete, the anagen phase starts and the new hair strand will push out the old hair strand. When this happens the old hair strand is shed. At any one time, 10% to 15% of your hair is in the telogen phase.

Factors That Are Stopping You From Getting Longer Hair

1. Dry hair

Just like a plant needs water to grow, our hair needs to be moisturized to grow. Due to its nature, our hair is already dry. Without getting the appropriate amount of moisture your hair becomes brittle and prone to breakage — stopping you from getting longer hair.

2. Excessive trimming

When it comes to trimming your hair, it should only be done with reason. A common myth is that trimming should be done on a regular schedule, but trimming when not necessary robs you of getting longer hair.

Trimming should be done to remove split ends and frayed hair. When you are trimming without any sign of damaged hair you are cutting off perfectly good hair.

3. Not trimming enough

On the flip side of excessive trimming is not trimming

enough. Trimming is a delicate balance between cutting off damaged hair and making sure you don't cut off hair in good condition. A visual check of your hair can tell you if you have split ends or frayed hair. Neglecting to cut off split ends will make the split travel up the hair shaft, leading to breakage and shorter hair.

4. Over processing

When your hair is over processed due to chemical relaxers or repeated coloring it is left dry, brittle and susceptible to breakage. A common cause of over processing hair is leaving relaxer in too long. You can avoid this by either having a good hairstylist apply the relaxer or if you decide to self-relax making sure you are sticking to the recommended times.

Another reason for over processing is combining chemical processes. Avoid coloring hair that has been relaxed and never relax hair that has been colored — it will lead to extreme breakage. If you do decide to color your hair, stick to natural dyes like Henna or color rinses.

5. Excessive Heat

When you are constantly applying heat to your hair it will dry out, becoming brittle and susceptible to breakage. Using a blow dryer or flat iron should be limited and should only be done on low to medium heat settings with a heat protectant having been applied to the hair.

6. Genetics

Genetics play a part in your hair growth. Genetics is not about being "mixed". Genetics are unique to each individual, even children of the same parents will have different sets of genes. Hair grows on average ½ an inch per month. What this means is that for some women hair grows less than ½ an inch per month and for some women hair grows more than ½ an inch per month. Whether you are below or above ½ an inch per month is determined by your genes.

Another way that genes affect hair growth is genetic hair loss. If there is pre-disposition to hair loss in the family, that will affect how long your hair can grow.

7. Applying grease to your scalp

For generations "greasing the scalp" has been considered good hair care that can make hair grow longer. Unfortunately, there is no scientific reason why this would work and it can actually be bad for your hair. When grease is applied to the scalp, it clogs the follicles and may lead to inflammation of the hair follicles causing hair loss.

8. Hair accessories

Misuse of hair accessories is an often overlooked source of breakage and damage to the hair. Hair can get caught in rubber bands and bobby pins. Also, when using rubber bands to hold a style, the hair can get pulled too tight.

To avoid these problems use Scrunchies or silk hair ties. Scrunchies and silk hair ties are less damaging to your hair. However, if you have no alternative but to use rubber bands, make sure to dip the rubber band in olive oil before putting it on your hair. With bobby pins make sure when you take them out — do it gently. Yanking bobby pins off your hair can lead to breakage.

9. Constant manipulation

Constant manipulation of the hair is another reason why many women fail to achieve their hair length goals. Hair needs to be given a rest. Constantly brushing, combing or changing your hairstyle every night is not good for your hair. The more you have combs, brushes and fingers running through your hair the more you increase the chances of breakage. Give your hair some rest if you want to achieve longer length.

10. Not protecting your hair while you sleep

Your hair needs to be protected while you sleep. When you go to sleep on a cotton pillow case, the cotton robs your hair of moisture and causes friction on your hair which leads to breakage.

The best way to protect your hair when sleeping is to wrap it up in silk/satin scarf or wear a silk/satin bonnet. If you find yourself forgetting to put on your scarf or bonnet before going to sleep, consider getting a silk/satin pillow case. Protecting your hair while you sleep will help you in achieving your hair length goals.

11. Stress

Stress affects hair growth and prevents many women from achieving their hair length goals. When your body is under constant stress, your body releases hormones that directly impact your hair follicles. When the stress is long term, it can lead to hair loss. There are a lot of things that can trigger stress from work to relationships. It becomes important to find ways to relieve stress like exercising and yoga.

12. Medication

Medication is another reason that could prevent you from achieving your hair length goals. Side effects from medication can alter the hair growth cycle to the point of accelerating shedding of the hair. If you have any concerns about the side effects of medication you are taking, discuss them with your physician.

13. Poor Diet

We are what we eat and a diet poor in nutrition can prevent

you from achieving your hair length goals. This doesn't mean you should only eat fruits and vegetables — it just means you should be mindful of what you are putting in your body if you want longer hair.

When your body is not getting enough nutrients, your hair suffers the most. To your body, hair is considered low in priority and not vital to your survival. Hair follicles will only get nutrients when other vital parts of your body have received sufficient nutrition. A diet that includes lots of water, dark green leafy vegetables, whole grains and meat in moderation is good for your body and your hair growth.

Factors That Help You Get Longer Hair

1. Moisturizing your hair

Your hair needs to be moisturized if it is to grow to any significant length. A good way to keep your hair moisturized is to spritz it with a water and glycerin mixture twice a day. Spritzing your hair replaces moisture lost to evaporation.

Besides spritzing your hair daily, you also want to moisturize your hair from the inside by drinking plenty of water. When your body is well hydrated, your hair is able to grow. Try and drink at least half your weight in ounces of water each day. Let's say you weigh 140 lbs, aim to drink around 70 oz of water every day.

2. Protective Styling

Protective styling helps you to grow your hair longer. A protective style is a hair style that protects the ends of your hair from friction and tension. A protective style should also keep your hair off your shoulders and clothing. A good protective style is one that is low maintenance and keeps the ends of your hair well protected.

3. Proper Detangling

Proper and regular detangling helps in the growth of your hair. Our hair's natural curl pattern makes it ideal for knots and tangles. If these knots and tangles are not detangled prior to handling your hair, they can lead to breakage.

When detangling on wash day, be patient with your knots and tangles. Give yourself enough time so you're not in a rush. It's easy to become frustrated with detangling but whenever you get to that point — remember proper detangling is a must if you are to have longer hair.

4. Scalp Massages

Massaging your scalp often (at least once a week) improves blood circulation at the hair follicles and relieves tension. Improved blood circulation at the scalp and stress relief are good for hair growth.

5. Keeping your scalp clean

In addition to scalp massages, you want to make sure your scalp is clean and clear of product build up. Unfortunately, there is a myth that has been passed around that a dirty scalp helps to grow your hair. This is just not true. A scalp that is free of product build up, dirt and dead skin cells is an environment where your hair can grow longer.

A dirty scalp means that your hair follicles become clogged and inflamed, which prevents you from achieving your hair length goal and can lead to hair loss.

6. Having a hair care regimen

Having a hair care regimen will help you grow longer hair. When no regimen is followed and your hair is neglected, you will suffer from unhealthy hair that will be prone to breakage. If you find that you're really busy with school or work and don't have time to follow a hair care regimen then go for a low maintenance hair style like braids or simplify your regimen.

7. Protein and Moisture balance

Your hair is mostly made up of protein and moisture (water). For it to grow long there must be a balance of protein and moisture maintained. Too little moisture leads to dry hair and breakage. Too little protein leads to weak hair that's prone to breakage. Too much moisture leads to limp hair and breakage. Too much protein leads to hard, brittle hair and breakage.

Using a protein conditioner or treatment when needed will repair damaged hair, maintaining a proper protein and moisture balance.

8. Nutrition

Your diet plays an important part in helping your hair grow. Our hair needs nutrients to grow and a diet lacking the right type of nutrients will stunt hair growth. A diet to make your hair grow long should include plenty of water and foods that have protein, vitamins A , B, C and E.

Foods that are also excellent for your hair include dark green leafy vegetables, wild caught salmon, walnuts, Brazilian nuts, avocados, eggs, turkey, Greek yoghurt, and beans. See the chapter *Healthy Hair Diet* for more suggestions.

9. Low manipulation

Low manipulation is important for your hair to grow longer. The less you're handling your hair, the less chances it will break due to handling. Low manipulation includes avoiding using brushes on your hair and if you must brush, do it slowly. Low manipulation also means having your hair in a protective style. Braids (that are not too tight!) are a good low manipulation hairstyle that allows your hair to grow long.

10. Patience

Patience is last on the list but is certainly not the least. When your goal is having longer hair, you have to realize it won't happen overnight. On average hair grows $1/2$ an inch per month and with no breakage at all, that works out to 6 inches a year. If you have just cut off all your hair that means it may take at least a couple of years to go past shoulder length.

The key is not to be discouraged along the way, just know that as long as you practice healthy hair care habits — you will get longer hair!

GROWING YOUR HAIR LONG

CHAPTER NINE

STRAIGHTENING YOUR HAIR

When it comes to straightening your hair, you will have the option of using a flat iron or a relaxer. Both work by altering the structure and bonds of your hair. Care should always be taken when using a flat iron or a relaxer.

Flat ironing your hair

Tips When Flat Ironing Your Hair

1. *Wash and deep condition*. Wash and deep condition your hair before using a flat iron. This removes product build up and moisturizes the hair. Allow your hair to fully dry before using a flat iron.

2. *Always use a heat protectant.* A heat protectant is a leave-in conditioner that slows down the transfer of heat from the flat iron to your hair, making the heat less damaging.

3. *Quality flat iron.* Use a high quality ceramic flat iron with an adjustable temperature dial not just a high-low switch. You want to know how much heat you are putting on your hair.

4. *Low temperature.* Use the lowest temperature setting that will get your hair straight. Work your way up the temperature rather than starting at the highest temperature. You don't want to use more heat than is necessary and end up burning your hair. Heat above **350° F** should be avoided.

5. *Flat iron in sections.* Divide your hair into smaller sections. It will make it easier for you as you flat iron and move from section to section.

6. *Flat ironing technique.* Flat iron from the roots to the ends. Limit to one pass, two at most.

7. *Sleeping.* When going to sleep, wrap your hair in a silk/satin scarf to prevent reversion and having to flat iron daily.

Relaxing your hair

Types of Relaxers

When it comes to relaxers you have two choices — no lye relaxer and lye relaxer. Let's go over the differences between the two.

Lye Relaxers

Lye relaxers contain sodium hydroxide as the main ingredient. A lye relaxer has a high pH range of between 12 to 14, allowing it to lift the cuticle and work much faster than a no lye relaxer. However, because of the high pH it can be very harsh — to the point of burning the scalp if left on for too long.

Lye relaxers are the relaxer of choice for professional hairstylists and ideally should only be used by someone with a good knowledge of how chemical relaxers work.

Advantages of a Lye Relaxer

- Doesn't leave mineral deposits on your hair like a no lye relaxer.
- Relaxes the hair faster than a no lye relaxer.
- Works very well for those with coarse hair. The high pH allows the cuticle to be lifted and have the relaxer go to work.
- It comes already mixed. No need to mix in an activator

Examples of popular lye relaxers: *Mizani , Silk Elements, Affirm.*

No Lye relaxers

No lye relaxers are relaxers that are meant for in-home use. A no lye relaxer can have *potassium hydroxide, lithium hydroxide or guanidine hydroxide* as the active ingredient. No Lye relaxers have a lower pH range (9 to 11) than lye relaxers (12 to 14) and will require more time to relax the hair.

While no lye relaxers are not as harsh on your scalp as lye relaxers, they will deposit minerals onto your hair. If these minerals are not washed off with chelating shampoo, your hair can become dry and brittle.

Advantages of a No Lye relaxer

- Good for those with a sensitive scalp.
- Since it can be left on the hair longer than lye relaxer, you can get much straighter hair.
- Easier to use if you are new to relaxing your own hair.
- Less expensive than a lye relaxer.

Tips on Self Relaxing

1. *Don't apply relaxer when you have broken skin.* If you scratch your scalp, wait at least a week before applying relaxer.

2. *Stick to the time on the box.* Never leave relaxer on your hair longer than the time that is recommended on the box. This tends to happen when you use a no lye relaxer, because a no lye relaxer does not have as much of a burning sensation like a lye relaxer. Remember, if you go past the recommended time you will be damaging your hair.

3. *Always follow up with a neutralizing shampoo.* If you do not follow up a relaxer with a neutralizing shampoo, the relaxer continues to work — breaking down the bonds in your hair. Neutralizing shampoo is designed to stop this process. For neutralizing shampoo to work best, leave it on your hair for a minimum of 6 to 8 minutes before rinsing it out.

4. *Always base your scalp.* Basing your scalp means applying petroleum jelly to your scalp to protect it from the harsh chemicals in the relaxer.

5. *Do not apply relaxer to previously relaxed hair.* When retouching, only apply relaxer to new growth. If you wait 8 to 10 weeks before retouching, you lower the chance of overlapping. You can also apply an oil to your relaxed hair to prevent overlapping. Olive oil and Castor oil work well for this purpose.

Tips on Maintaining Relaxed Hair

1 . *Deep condition regularly.* Deep conditioning moisturizes your hair and restores its "condition". Aim to deep condition at least once or twice a month.

2. *Use a temporary color or color rinse.* If you decide to color your relaxed hair, it is best for your hair to use a color rinse. A color rinse is the least damaging dye to your relaxed hair.

3. *Limit heat.* Whenever you relax your hair it becomes weakened. Excessive heat will dry out your hair. A combination of weak and dry hair will lead to breakage. Limit heat and always use a heat protectant.

4. *Trim split ends.* Make sure you are cutting off split ends. If you delay in cutting off split ends they will travel up the hair shaft causing more damage to your hair.

5. *Protect your hair when sleeping.* To protect your relaxed hair from damage when sleeping, sleep on a silk/satin pillowcase or wrap your hair with a silk/satin scarf.

6. *Limit shampooing.* Shampoo contains ingredients called sulfates that strip your hair of its natural oils. Limit shampooing to once or twice a month. In place of shampooing, you should conditioner wash (co-wash).

7. *Keep your relaxed hair moisturized.* Your hair needs moisture. This is done by using a moisturizing conditioner on wash day and moisturizing daily with a daily moisturizer of your choice.

8. *Do a protein treatment but don't overdo it.* A protein treatment will strengthen and repair damaged hair. A protein treatment should be done no more than once every 6 to 8 weeks.

9. *Stretch your relaxer.* Instead of relaxing your hair every 4 to 6 weeks, try and extend it to 8 to 10 weeks. By "stretching" you decrease the chance of overlapping relaxer and over processing your hair.

CHAPTER TEN

WEAVES AND WIGS

You may have at one point found yourself thinking should I wear a weave or a wig ? Weaves and wigs are excellent styling options but they serve different purposes. This chapter will go over weaves and wigs.

Weave and Wig terms to know

To help you better understand the world of weave and wig buying, below is a guide to the terms used:

Virgin hair : Virgin hair is high quality human hair that has the cuticles intact and running in the same direction. Virgin hair has not been altered or chemically processed in any way.

Remy or Remi hair : Remy hair is high quality human hair that has the cuticles intact and running in the same direction. The benefit of having the cuticles run in the same direction is that the hair is not easily tangled, making it easier to manage. Remy hair has been processed by adding either color or perm.

Non-Remy hair : Non-remy hair is lower quality human hair. The cuticles do not run in the same direction, meaning the roots and ends are mixed up. When the cuticles do not run in the same direction, the likelihood of knots and tangles increases.

Non-remy hair has been chemically processed and is the weave hair more commonly found in beauty supply stores. Non-remy hair does not last as long as Virgin or Remy hair.

Single drawn hair : Single drawn hair is hair from a single donor. Single drawn hair contains hair of different lengths, combining both long and short lengths — just as it was on the donor's head. When you buy single drawn hair it will have a range of length e.g. 10 - 12 inches.

Double drawn : Double drawn hair is hair that has been obtained from multiple donors. Double drawn hair is all of the same length. The 'double-drawn' refers to the process of having the hair go through a process of machine sorting and then going through a second process of hand sorting to get hair of the same length. When you buy double drawn hair it will have the same length e.g. 18 inches.

Brazilian hair : Hair sold as Brazilian hair is silky and soft in texture. It blends easier with relaxed hair. Brazilian hair will hold curls well. Brazilian hair from Brazil is rare and hard to find . What you will often get is Indian hair that has been processed and is marketed as "Brazilian Hair".

Indian Hair : Indian hair is the most popular weave hair. You can see the process of how Indian hair is obtained in Chris Rock's movie *Good Hair*. Women donate their hair to the religious temples where it's then sold to the highest bidder, processed and shipped to America.

Indian hair is a good match for relaxed hair and holds curls well.

Chinese hair : Chinese hair is the most commonly found human hair and also the least expensive. When you go to a beauty supply store, you are more than likely buying Chinese hair. Chinese hair is bone straight and does not hold curls well.

Pros to wearing a weave:

1. *As a protective hair style.* A weave can be worn while transitioning from relaxed to natural hair.

2. *Expand your styling options.* You can straighten or curl a high quality weave.

3. *Less damage to your own hair.* You can apply heat or color to a weave without having to worry about damaging your own hair.

4. *You can achieve instant length.* Weaves are great for adding length to your hair.

Cons to wearing a weave:

1. *Hair loss.* Weaves can lead to hair loss if the braiding is done too tight.

2. *Expensive.* Quality weaves can be costly running into the thousands of dollars for both the hair itself and the cost of the install.

3. *A bird's nest*. Using low quality weave hair and improper weave care can leave your hair looking like a " bird's nest".

4. *Neglecting your own hair*. Neglect of your own hair underneath the weave can lead to dry, damaged hair.

Pros to wearing a wig:

1. *Saves time*. You can change your hairstyle instantly without having to book an appointment at the salon and sit for hours getting your hair done.

2. *Multiple Options*. You have multiple styling options. You're are not limited to one style. You can take off the wig and wear your hair natural.

3. *Less strain on your hair*. Wigs place less strain on your hair when compared to weaves that require braiding.

4. *Easier maintenance*. Wigs are easier to maintain because they can be taken off easily, detangled, washed and styled.

5. *Gray hair and balding spots*. Wigs are an excellent option to cover gray hair or balding spots.

Cons to wearing a wig:

1. *Expensive*. High quality wigs can be costly running into the several thousands of dollars for a custom lace wig.

2. *Hot in the summer*. Wigs can get hot especially in the summer and quickly get very uncomfortable to wear.

3. *Can be blown away by the wind*. When you compare weaves to wigs, wigs that are not properly fitted can be blown away by the wind creating an embarrassing situation.

What to consider before buying weave hair or a wig

When it comes to buying weave hair, there are several questions you want to ask yourself so you can get the best out of your purchase. These questions also apply when buying a wig. Before you make the purchase, ask yourself:

1. *Do I want human hair or synthetic hair?*

You can color, straighten or curl human hair. You cannot do the same with synthetic hair. If you plan on coloring, flat ironing or curling then you should go for human hair.

2. *Does it match my hair texture?*

When buying weave hair you want to match your own hair texture as much as possible. Weave hair that closely matches your hair texture will blend in with your own hair and seem more natural.

3. *How much am I willing to spend?*

When it comes to weaves and wigs, the old saying "you get what you pay for" applies. In general, as the price goes up so does the quality. Higher quality weave hair will tend to last longer than lower quality weave hair.

4. *Will I be using heat?*

If you intend to use a flat or curling iron then you will need to buy human hair. Synthetic hair is made of plastic and will melt as you apply heat.

5. *Do I want curly or straight?*

For the most part, you will have more styling options, easier maintenance and a more natural look with a curly weave.

6. *How long do I intend to wear my weave?*

If you intend to wear your weave for more than a month then you will need to go for human hair. High quality human hair weave can last several installs.

7 .*Will I be coloring the weave?*

If you intend to color your weave, go with human hair. You cannot color synthetic hair.

8. *Will I be swimming?*

Quality human hair weaves will do fine if you go swimming. However, low quality synthetic hair may get tangled if you go swimming. Buy quality human weave hair if you will be swimming often.

Tips on Wearing and Maintaining Weaves

1. *Buy the highest quality weave hair you can afford.*

Synthetic hair at the beauty supply store might be appealing because of its lower price but it limits you to what you can do. This does not mean you should spend an exorbitant amount to buy your weave hair, this means with weave hair you get what you pay for.

2. *Make sure your own hair is in good condition.* Before getting your weave install, you want to make sure your own hair is in good condition. Detangle, wash, condition and moisturize your own hair before the install. Also cut off any split ends.

3. *Get rid of factory smells and chemicals.* Before your weave install, co-wash your weave hair to remove factory smells and any chemicals that may irritate your scalp. Allow your weave hair to fully dry before you do your install.

4. *Get a good hairstylist for the install.* Get a hairstylist who is well reviewed to install your weave. You don't want to spend a lot of money on your weave hair and then have a hairstylist do a bad job.

5. *Make sure your braids are not too tight.* Let the hairstylist know if you feel any pain or discomfort. Tight

braids under the weave will cause you to have constant headaches from the pulling and can eventually lead to permanent hair loss.

6. *Treat your weave like it's your own hair.* After the install, you want to start treating the weave like it's your own hair. This means having a hair care regimen in place. This means detangling, washing and conditioning the weave. Having a regimen will make your weave stay fresh and last longer.

7. *Don't keep your weave for too long.* You don't want to go longer than 8 weeks. Ideally you should wear a weave for about 6 weeks or less. Removing the weave gives your own hair a break. It also gives you a chance to properly wash and condition your own hair.

Tips to buying your weave hair online

Buying weave hair online is now pretty common. Vendors are often in foreign countries and it may be difficult to get a refund if the transaction goes wrong. Follow these tips to ensure that you get what you're paying for:

1. *Google search.* Do a Google search of the company you are buying from. Unfortunately, you can't trust every company selling weave hair online. Check out the reviews by typing into the Google search bar — the name of the company and the word "review" or "reviews".

2. *YouTube reviews.* A lot of YouTube reviews are paid reviews or the person reviewing the hair was sent the hair at no cost and has an incentive to give a positive review. The most reliable reviews are when the person used their own money to buy the hair.

3. *Brazilian hair.* Be careful when buying hair that is being sold as "Brazilian hair". Brazilian hair is rare. A lot of companies just sell Indian hair that has been processed and packaged as "Brazilian hair".

4. *Too good a price.* If the price is too good to be true then it probably is. If you find a company selling Virgin or Remy hair for a significantly lower price than other vendors, you will want to proceed with caution and make sure the company is actually legit.

5. *Contact.* Contact the vendor before you make your

purchase . This allows you to get any questions you may have answered and also gives you an opportunity to see how good a response / customer service the company has.

Tips on sleeping while wearing a weave

1. *You want to protect your weave while you're sleeping to prevent matting and tangling*:

For straight weaves: You can sleep on a silk/satin pillowcase or wrap the weave under a silk/satin scarf.

For curly or wavy weave: Detangle the weave first, section it into two or more braids and then wrap it under a silk/satin scarf.

2. *Make sure you never go to sleep with wet hair.* Wet hair allows bacteria to grow which leads to mildew smell coming from the weave. Make sure your hair is dry before going to sleep.

Tips on swimming while wearing a weave

1. *It's ok to go swimming with your weave.* Remi and

Virgin hair are better able to with stand water. Synthetic and lower quality hair may matte and tangle after swimming.

2. *Soak your weave with fresh tap water before going into the pool.* By wetting your weave, the water will act as a barrier preventing your weave from absorbing the chlorine filled water.

3. *After swimming.* Immediately after swimming, rinse out your weave with fresh tap water.

4. *Shampoo and condition you weave.* You will need to use a clarifying or swimmers shampoo to remove the chlorine.

Tips on exercising while wearing a weave

1. *Put your weave up in a high ponytail or bun.* This will prevent sweat from getting to your weave.

2. *Wear a sweat headband.* The headband will absorb most of the sweat as you work out. A good headband is the Dri-sweat Edge women's headband (available on Amazon.com).

3. *After work out.* After your work out, co-wash and use a leave-in conditioner to keep your weave looking and smelling fresh.

Weave Problems and Remedies

1. Itchy scalp when wearing a weave

An itchy scalp is common among weave wearers. Whenever your scalp itches, it's a way of your scalp telling you something is wrong.

Causes:

- Allergic reaction to chemicals used when the weave hair was being processed.
- Product build up that's clogging up the pores on the scalp.
- Fungal growth on the scalp causing dandruff.

Prevention :

- Wash your weave hair before an install to remove any chemicals that might cause an allergic reaction.
- Keep your scalp moisturized when wearing a weave. Hot oil treatments are a good way to keep your scalp moisturized.

Remedies :

- *Anti-dandruff shampoo.* Anti-dandruff shampoo prevents fungal growth and removes the dandruff.
- *Witch Hazel.* Witch hazel is a powerful natural astringent and will help soothe the scalp. You can dip a cotton swab in the witch hazel and gently dab into where the scalp itches.
- *Tea tree oil.* Add a few drops of tea tree oil to your regular shampoo. Tea tree oil has antifungal properties and prevents growth of fungus on the scalp.
- *Dermatologist.* If your scalp continues to itch after you have tried different remedies, you will want to consult a dermatologist.

2. Mildew / Musty / Bad smells from a weave

Causes:

- When the hair underneath the weave is left wet after a wash, bacteria and mildew begin to grow which causes an odor.
- Product build up on the scalp.

Prevention:

- Make sure the hair underneath the weave is thoroughly dry after a wash. If time and the weather permits you can air dry, if not use a blow dryer on low to medium setting or sit under a hooded dryer.

- Remove product build up with a shampoo. Make sure to focus on the scalp when shampooing.

CHAPTER ELEVEN

COLORING YOUR HAIR

Coloring your hair is an excellent way to get a different and stylish look. When it comes to coloring your hair, you have several options and it's important to know what those options are and what they do for your hair.

You have the option of using a temporary color, a semi-permanent color, a demi-permanent or a permanent color. You also have the option of using a synthetic dye or a natural dye.

The Different Types of Colors

Temporary Color : A temporary color or color rinse will wash off after your first shampoo wash. A temporary color is a good option for one off events like weddings or graduations. Temporary color is the least damaging option when coloring your hair. A temporary color will coat the cuticle instead of entering the hair shaft.

Semi-Permanent Color : A semi-permanent color will usually last between 6 to 12 shampoo washes. A semi-permanent color does not contain ammonia or peroxide and cannot lighten your hair.

Demi-Permanent Color : A demi-permanent color is very much like a semi-permanent color but will last a little longer, usually between 12 to 26 shampoo washes.

Permanent Color : Permanent color as the name implies is permanent and cannot be washed off. The only way to remove permanent color is to cut off the color treated hair. Permanent color contains both ammonia and peroxide and works by penetrating inside the hair shaft. Permanent color is a good option if you want to dye graying hair.

Natural Dyes and Synthetic Dyes

The difference between natural and synthetic dyes is that natural dyes are made from plants and synthetic dyes are made in a laboratory. Natural dyes have been in use for thousands of years, while synthetic dyes are a recent discovery. Synthetic dyes have become popular because of their low cost and promotion from dye manufacturers.

In general, synthetic dyes are more likely to damage the hair, irritate the scalp and cause allergic reactions when compared to natural dyes. If you have the option to use a synthetic dye or a natural dye, go for the natural dye — it is better for your hair.

Natural Dyes - Henna, Indigo and Cassia Obvata

Henna : Henna is made from the leaves of the plant, *Lawsonia Inermis*. Henna dye comes in powder form and will color your hair a reddish color. Different colors can be achieved by mixing henna with other natural dyes. When purchasing henna, you want to purchase Body Art Quality (BAQ) henna. BAQ henna is the purest and most concentrated form of henna.

Besides coloring your hair, henna is known to improve its condition. It can make your hair *stronger* and *silkier*. A disadvantage to henna is that it can be very difficult to apply by yourself. Proper care must taken when applying henna because it can permanently stain your clothes, bed sheets and pillow case. If you are new to henna it is best to get a professional hairstylist to do it or have a friend help you out.

Indigo : Indigo is a dye derived from the plant *Indigofera Tinctoria*. Indigo is a deep blue dye and is often mixed with henna for a brownish color. Indigo comes in powder form and has a strong, distinctive fresh peas smell.

Cassia Obovata : Cassia Obovata is more commonly referred to as senna or cassia. It is a dye derived from the leaves of the *Cassia Obovata* plant. Cassia is known to improve the condition and shine of the hair. Cassia will not add color to dark colored hair but can add a golden yellow color to gray hair.

Tips for Coloring Relaxed Hair

1. *You can color relaxed hair but never relax hair that's been colored.* Relaxing hair that has been colored is extremely damaging to the hair.

2. *When coloring relaxed hair, it is best to use a temporary color or color rinse.* These are less damaging to the hair.

3. *If you're not sure what you are doing don't try and color your own hair.* Get a professional to do it. Synthetic dyes are chemicals and can be damaging to your scalp and hair.

4. *Avoid swimming when your hair has been color treated.* Chlorine in the water can mix with chemicals from the dye, which can be damaging to your hair.

5. *When you use synthetic dyes on relaxed hair, you are further weakening your hair.* Proper maintenance and conditioning is required to prevent dry hair and breakage.

Tips for Coloring Natural Hair

1. *Stick to natural dyes like henna.* Using synthetic dyes is similar to using a relaxer. Synthetic dyes will weaken and dry your hair.

2. *If you decide to use a synthetic dye, use a color rinse.* It will cause the least damage.

3. *Never bleach your natural hair.* It is very damaging to the hair.

4. *Follow your regimen.* Continue to follow your hair care regimen, conditioning and moisturizing your hair.

Tips for Coloring Weaves and Wigs

1. *Experiment.* Weaves and wigs are a great way to experiment with color and not have to worry about damaging your own hair.

2. *Color before install.* While you can color your weave after the install, it is best to color it *before* the install. Coloring the weave after the install adds an extra level of difficulty (and a chance to mess things up) that could have been avoided.

3. *Quality human hair.* If you are planning on coloring your weave or wig, make sure you get quality human hair. You cannot add color to synthetic hair.

CHAPTER TWELVE

COMMON HAIR PROBLEMS AND REMEDIES

This chapter will go over how to prevent and remedy common hair problems. The common hair problems will go over are:

1. Excessive dandruff.
2. Chronically dry hair.
3. Breakage
4. Split ends
5. Traction Alopecia
6. Excessive hair shedding
7. Knots and tangles

1. Excessive Dandruff

What is it?

Dandruff is a condition where dead skin cells are shed from the scalp. Dandruff is a normal body process but when dandruff becomes excessive it is a sign of a bigger, underlying problem.

Causes:

1. Allergic reaction to hair products. Certain hair products contain ingredients that can irritate the scalp.

2. Not shampooing often enough. Shampooing removes product build up and dead skin cells from the scalp.

3. Stress. Chronic stress can trigger excessive dandruff.

4. Over consumption of sugary and processed foods.

5. Production of a fungus on the scalp called *Malassezia*.

6. Seborrhoeic dermatitis, Psoriasis and Eczema. All conditions of the skin that would have to be diagnosed by a

dermatologist.

Prevention:

1. Shampooing your hair to remove build up.

2. Eating a diet low in sugars and processed foods.

3. Relieving stress through exercise.

Remedies:

1. Anti-dandruff shampoo.

2. Apple Cider Vinegar rinse.

3. Visit a dermatologist to see if there is an underlying skin condition.

2. Chronically Dry hair

Causes:

1. Excessive use of shampoos. Shampoo contains

ingredients called sulfates that strip the hair of its natural oils.

2. High porosity hair due to damaged cuticles. When you have high porosity hair, it has the ability to absorb moisture but quickly loses the moisture as well.

3. Excessive use of heat. Excessive use of flat irons and blow dryers on a high setting will dry the hair.

4. Alcohol. Using hair products that contain certain alcohols that have a drying effect on the hair.

5. Not drinking enough water. Your body and hair is hydrated from the water you drink. If you are not drinking enough water your hair will suffer. (Ideally drink at least half your body weight in ounces of water per day).

6. Not sealing in moisture. After you have moisturized your hair, you must follow up by sealing with an oil or butter to prevent moisture loss.

7. Not deep conditioning often enough. Use of a moisturizing deep conditioner at the very least once a

month.

Prevention:

1. Limit use of shampoo to once or twice a month.

2. Limit or avoid use of heat. If using heat, use a heat protectant.

3. Check hair products for alcohols like *isopropyl alcohol* and *ethyl alcohol* which are drying to the hair.

4. Drink plenty of water.

5. Use an oil or butter to seal in moisture.

Remedies:

1. Deep conditioning often. Deep condition with a moisturizing conditioner at least once or twice a month.

2. Try the L.O.C, L.C.O, L.C.S.O or Baggy methods of keeping hair moisturized.

3. Spritz your hair with a water and glycerin mix daily.

3. Breakage

Causes:

1. Lack of moisture. Your hair needs water, when it is not moisturized on a regular basis (spritzing daily and conditioning) it becomes brittle and more likely to break when combing.

2. Not protecting your ends. Your ends are the oldest part of your hair and require extra protection and care. Friction from clothing (also scarves) will cause your hair to break.

3. Constant manipulation. Frequent brushing and combing of your hair can cause breakage.

4. Knots and tangles. The kinky, coily nature of our hair makes it a breeding ground for knots and tangles.

5. Over processing. Overuse of chemicals, hair coloring and heat all weaken your hair. Once weakened your hair becomes easier to break.

6. Towel drying hair. The rubbing force caused by towel drying can damage your hair and lead to breakage.

7. Blow drying your hair. Pay attention to never completely dry your hair with a blow dryer. Leave a little moisture and let it air dry.

8. Leaving relaxer in for too long. When you self relax or your hairstylist leaves in the relaxer more than the recommend time, your hair is weakened. If you experience breakage right after relaxing, this could be the cause.

9. Excessive heat. Heat has a drying effect on the hair, making it brittle and prone to breakage.

10. Not protecting your hair when you sleep. Friction and rubbing against a cotton pillowcase can cause breakage.

Prevention:

1. Moisturize your hair daily by spritzing with a water and glycerin mix.

2. Wear protective styles. Protective styles are hair styles that protect your ends from tension and friction.

3. Use a plastic wide tooth comb when combing or detangling.

4. Minimize heat. Minimize or avoid using a flat iron and a blow dryer.

5. Have a proper balance of moisture and protein.

6. If you want to color your hair, choose a natural dye like henna or a color rinse.

7. Get a satin/silk pillowcase or bonnet to protect your hair when sleeping. Satin and silk are gentler on your hair.

4. Split ends

Causes:

1. Over processing your hair. Excessive use of heat, hair coloring and chemical treatments.

2. Excessive combing and brushing of the hair.

Prevention:

1. Avoid or minimize heat on your hair.

2. Regular deep conditioning.

3. Daily spritzing of your hair, paying special attention to the ends.

4. Low manipulation. Wear your hair in protective styles and avoid use of brushes.

Remedy:

Split ends cannot be fixed. Once they appear, you will need to cut them off.

5. Traction Alopecia

Causes:

1 .Traction alopecia is hair loss caused by constant pulling to the hair. Hair loss occurs along the hair line — with the temples and sides of the head being the most affected. Tight braids and sew-in weaves are major causes of traction alopecia.

Prevention:

1 . Avoid wearing hairstyles that place unnecessary tension on your head. Always make sure when you get braids or a sew-in weave, the braids are not too tight.

2. Wear hairstyles that are gentler on your hair like twist outs and bantu knots.

Remedies:

1. Traction alopecia comes in two forms — reversible and non reversible. Reversible traction alopecia can be cured by resting your hair and allowing the hair to grow back. Using

medications like *Minoxidil* can also help.

2. Non reversible traction alopecia, like the name implies, cannot be reversed. The hair loss is permanent because of permanent damage to the hair follicle, which is why you want to pay careful attention to hair loss in its early stages to prevent non reversible traction alopecia.

6. Excessive Hair Shedding

Causes:

Hair shedding is a normal part of the hair growth cycle. When a hair strand comes to the end of its life cycle, it is shed. If you find that you are shedding more hair than is normal for you then the causes could be :

1. Hormones: Change in hormones after giving birth can lead to excessive shedding.

2. Medication: Several medications including those taken for blood pressure, birth control and chemotherapy can lead to excessive hair shedding.

3. Stress: When you are under chronic stress, shedding can increase.

Prevention:

1. If you notice an increase in shedding, it is best to contact your physician to narrow down the cause.

7. Knots and Tangles

Cause:

1. Due to its unique curl pattern our hair is more likely to knot and tangle.

2. Shedding hair also increases knots and tangles.

Prevention:

1. Regular finger and wide tooth comb detangling.

2. Washing your hair regularly to remove shed hair.

3. Keep your hair moisturized. Dry hair is more likely to

knot and tangle.

CHAPTER THIRTEEN

DEALING WITH WINTER AND SUMMER

Weather poses a unique challenge to Black hair. If your hair is not properly protected during times of extreme cold or hot weather it can dry out, become damaged and eventually lead to breakage. You will need a plan on how to take care of your hair during times of extreme weather.

Dealing with Winter weather

The cold weather will cause your hair to dry out and become brittle. For thousands of years Black people lived in the warm climates of Africa. Our bodies (and hair) adapted to a warm and sunny environment. Our hair as people of African descent was never suited for extreme cold weather. Over the centuries due to slavery and migration black people can now be found in some of the coldest parts of the world.

With winter weather you will need to know how to protect your hair inside the house as well as outside the house.

Tips to dealing with your hair outside the house during winter

1. *Wear a hat.* Wear a hat to cover and protect your hair from the cold when you step outside. Avoid wool hats as they can cause rubbing and friction to your hair. Choose a hat with a satin/silk lining.

2. *Make sure your hair is dry.* If it's your wash day, make sure your hair has dried before you go outside. Never go outside in the cold weather with wet hair.

3. *Friction from a coat.* When wearing a coat, avoid coats that are made of a rough material. The rough material can catch your ends causing breakage. You can wear a silk scarf to protect your ends when wearing a coat.

4. *Stay hydrated.* Drink plenty of water. Water hydrates both your body and your hair.

Tips to dealing with your hair inside the house during winter

1. *Central heating can be drying to your hair.* Keep your hair moisturized by spritzing your hair when you are inside.

2. *Leave-in conditioner.* Use a leave-in conditioner on wash day to keep your hair moisturized.

3. *Keep your hair wrapped up.* Keep your hair wrapped up in a silk/satin scarf. This will keep the moisture locked in and when going to sleep it will prevent friction and rubbing against your pillow.

4. *Avoid coloring your hair during winter.* Synthetic dyes have a drying effect on your hair. Coloring your hair during the winter further dries out your hair.

5. *Stay hydrated.* Drinking water keeps both your body and hair hydrated.

Great hairstyles for the winter

Below is a list of hairstyles that are great for protecting your hair during the winter. Not only do they protect your hair from the cold, windy weather but they protect your hair from friction and rubbing against coats and cotton scarves:

1. Braids (*make sure your braids are not too tight!*)
2. Wigs
3. Sew-in weaves
4. Updos
5. Buns

Dealing with Summer weather

While winter is about protecting your hair from the frigid cold and the wind, summer is about protecting your hair from the drying heat and damaging ultraviolet (UV) rays from sun. In the summer you also have to protect your hair from sea salt and chlorine if you swim.

Tips to dealing with your hair outside the house during summer

1. *Wear a hat.* If you are going to be in the sun for long periods of time, protect your hair by wearing a hat. Straw hats and even baseball caps can do a good job of protecting your hair from the sun.

2. *Drink water.* The summer can be extremely drying to your hair. Drink plenty of water to hydrate your body and hair.

3. *Silk or satin scarf.* You can also wear a silk or satin scarf wrapped around your hair to protect it from the sun.

Tips to dealing with your hair inside the house during summer

1. *Stay hydrated.* Keep your body and hair hydrated by drinking plenty of water.

2. *Spritz often.* Spritz your hair frequently to keep it

moisturized.

Great hairstyles for the summer

Below is a list of hairstyles that are great at protecting your hair from the summer heat and UV rays. They also protect your ends from breakage.

1. Box braids
2. Sew-in weave
3. Micro braids
4. Twists

CHAPTER FOURTEEN

BABY, TODDLER AND PRE-TEEN HAIR

When taking care of children's hair, two things to always remember are to be gentle with their hair and the less done to their hair the better. Unfortunately, most women are never taught how to properly take of their baby's hair and end up using the same hair care practices and products they use for their own hair. This chapter will help you take care of your child's hair.

Tips for Newborn to 2 years

1. *The first 6 months.* During her first 6 months, you will want to avoid using hair products with chemicals on your

baby's hair.

Not only is it not necessary at this stage but at this point you don't know if your baby is allergic to certain chemicals found in hair products. For the most part, gently rinsing the baby's hair with luke warm water should be enough to wash her hair.

2. *Be extra gentle with her hair.* When handling her hair be extra gentle when washing or brushing it.

3. *No finger nails.* When washing her hair, use the pads of your fingers to remove any dirt or food that may be on her scalp and hair. Using your finger nails might scratch her tender scalp and lead to infection of the broken skin.

4. *Get her used to your hands in her hair.* During the first couple years you want to get her used to your hands washing and styling her hair. By doing this, you can prevent future hair washing and styling battles as she gets older — especially around the 2 to 3 year mark.

Often the cause of these battles is a bad experience that she had with shampoo getting in her eye or her hair being pulled roughly by a brush.

5. *Keep her hair moisturized.* As her hair grows, you want to keep it moisturized. After washing her hair, you can use a 'baby' leave in conditioner that is chemical free and does not contain any scalp irritating ingredients. A good baby hair conditioner is *California Baby Hair Conditioner.* You can also spritz her hair with a water and glycerin mix for keeping the hair moisturized daily.

6. *Good hair styles.* Good hair styles at this age are just simply having her wear a cute headband, pigtails or ponytails.

7. *Avoid beads.* At this age you want to avoid hair styles with beads. Beads can be a choking hazard for infants.

Toddler and Pre-Teen (3 years to 12 years)

1. *Hair care regimen.* Now is a good time to start a regular hair care regimen that involves detangling, washing, conditioning and daily moisturizing of her hair.

2. *Explain as you go along.* As she gets older, she will be curious as to why you do certain things to her hair. This is a

good time to start teaching her about healthy hair care practices.

3. *Develop a positive self image.* Build in her a positive self image about her natural hair. At this age, she will watch TV and see women who have hair that doesn't look like her own. It is important you let her know that there is nothing wrong with her hair being different. Let her know she has beautiful hair and show her pictures of celebrities who have hair like her own.

At this age you also want to avoid saying things that will damage her self-image. Saying things like "Your hair is so difficult" or "You have bad hair" will create a lifelong impression and she will grow up thinking that there is something wrong with her natural hair.

4. *Hair accessories.* At this age beads and other hair accessories are fine. Just make sure that any hair accessories you use do not snag or cause breakage.

5. *Protecting her hair while sleeping.* For protecting her hair while she sleeps you can use a silk or satin pillowcase. This is a better option than wrapping with a scarf because young children will likely pull off any scarf or bonnet as they

sleep. As she gets older and gets used to sleeping with something on her hair, you can use a silk/satin scarf or bonnet.

6. *Styling options*. Great styling options at this age are braids (not too tight), buns, pony tails and twists.

7. *Swimming*. When she swims make sure her hair is protected with a swimming cap. Use a clarifying shampoo and a conditioner after swimming.

8. *Trim*. At this age she will start having split ends and frayed hair. To prevent the damage travelling further up the hair shaft, cut off the split ends.

9. *Avoid relaxing her hair*. Relaxing hair at a young age is never a good idea. Without proper care and frequent touch ups this can lead to damaged hair and breakage. In addition, the long term effect of the chemicals in relaxers on young girls is not yet fully known. Studies have linked using relaxers to fibroid tumors and even the 'kiddie relaxers' contain the same type of chemicals as the regular relaxers.

CHAPTER FIFTEEN

HEALTHY HAIR DIET

What you eat is directly related to the condition of your hair. Our hair relies on nutrients to grow healthy and strong. A diet lacking in nutritious food leads to unhealthy, weak hair.

You Hair Comes Last

When it comes to bodily functions your hair is last in line to receive nutrition. Your body will first distribute all the nutrients that are available to your vital organs. If there are any leftover nutrients, they are then sent to your hair. This is why it is important to eat a nutritious diet because if your diet is lacking in nutrition, your hair will get no nutrients. If you find that you're following a hair care regimen but your hair looks limp and lifeless, it could be down to a bad diet.

So what should you include in your diet to have

healthy hair? This chapter will go over the foods, vitamins and "super foods" that will help you to have healthy, beautiful hair.

Foods that are great for your hair

Water

Water is the number one thing that you should include in your diet. No other drink no matter what it says on the bottle can replace water. Water moisturizes your hair from the inside and is essential for hair growth. Aim to drink half of your body weight in ounces of water per day. Let's say you weigh 140 lbs, aim to drink 70 ounces of water each day to help hair growth and body metabolism.

Wheatgrass Juice

Wheatgrass is considered a "superfood" because it is densely packed with nutrients. As an added bonus, wheat grass is an excellent appetite suppressant for those trying to lose weight. Wheatgrass contains about 90 minerals, 20 amino acids (the stuff your hair is made of !) and is rich in vitamins.

There are several ways to consume wheatgrass. A popular method is to use a juicer to juice fresh wheatgrass. Another method is to make a shake or smoothie out of wheatgrass. Wheatgrass does have a bitter, distinctive taste that is why it's mostly taken as shots rather than as a full glass.

Moringa

Moringa is another "superfood" that is densely packed with nutrients that are excellent for your hair. Native to northwestern India, you can buy it online from places like Amazon.com in either powder form or capsules. *Moringa has tremendous benefits to the hair.* Per ounce, Moringa has 4 times more beta-carotene than carrots, 7 times more Vitamin C than orange juice, 3 times more iron than almonds, 4 times more calcium than milk and 2 times more protein than milk. Moringa is known to promote hair growth, reduce the production of dandruff and reverse hair loss.

Note: Moringa <u>SHOULD NOT</u> be taken by pregnant women as it can cause complications.

Dark Green Leafy Vegetables

Dark green leafy vegetables are good for your hair because they assist in the production of sebum — which lubricates your hair. Hair that is lacking in sebum is dry, brittle and can easily break off. Dark green leafy vegetables also contain Vitamins A and C. Examples of dark green leafy vegetables are spinach, kale and broccoli.

Foods Rich in Protein

Your hair is made of up to 90% protein. Protein gives your hair its strength. Hair that is lacking in protein is weak, has slow growth and can easily break off. Foods that are rich in protein include eggs, poultry and beans.

Nuts

Nuts are also good for your hair. Two types of nuts are best - walnuts and Brazilian nuts. Walnuts have an Omega-3 fatty acid called *alpha-linolenic acid*. The benefits of alpha-linolenic acid include providing nutrition directly to your hair follicles and can help in stopping hair loss. Brazilian Nuts contain *selenium*. Selenium helps in the growth of your hair. Selenium also has anti-fungal properties and prevents excessive dandruff.

Vitamins / Vitamin Supplements

While you can get most of your vitamin needs from the food you eat, there may be times like during winter when you need to take vitamin supplements. The following vitamins are all good for your hair and can be found in eggs, carrots, whole grains, wild caught salmon, milk, peas and lentils:

Vitamin B1 (thiamine)

Vitamin B2

Vitamin B3

Vitamin B5 (pantothenic acid)

Vitamin B6

Vitamin B7 (biotin)

Vitamin B9

Vitamin B12

This group of vitamins is commonly referred to as the B-complex vitamins.

A note on exercising

Exercising is not only good for your body but it's also good for your hair. One of the most common causes of hair loss and graying is stress. By exercising regularly, you help to reduce the levels of body stress hormones.

A note on dieting

While dieting to lose weight can be a good idea, pay careful attention that you are not starving your hair of much needed nutrients. Some diets while effective at making you lose weight, deny the body of much needed nutrients which can affect your hair growth. If you start a diet and you notice a difference in your hair — it could be due to a nutrient deficiency. Taking supplements and eating vegetables is one way around this while you are on a diet.

CHAPTER SIXTEEN

CLOSING WORDS

The purpose of this book was to give you a better understanding of how to take care of your hair. Hair care is a lifelong commitment and it is my hope that you will continue practicing healthy hair care habits.

I would love to hear your thoughts on the book. You can send me an email at lisajohnsonauthor@yahoo.com.

Best wishes on your hair journey,

Lisa Johnson
February 2014
Columbus, Ohio

BONUSES

HOW TO MAKE YOUR OWN SHAMPOO AND CONDITIONER

When you make your own shampoo and conditioner you know which ingredients exactly you're putting in your hair and you can avoid the harsh chemicals often found in commercial products. Making your own hair products also allows you to add your own unique twist.

Shampoos

1. Baking Soda Shampoo

Ingredients (for 1 time use)

1 Tbsp baking soda
1 Cup warm water

Directions

Mix baking soda and water in a small bottle and shake well.

Apply to hair and scalp. Gently massage scalp for 1 to 2 minutes to remove product build up and dirt. Rinse out with water.

Because baking soda shampoo is strongly alkaline and lifts the cuticle, follow it up with an apple cider vinegar rinse. The apple cider vinegar rinse will close the cuticles and add shine to the hair.

Apple Cider Vinegar (ACV) Rinse

Ingredients (for 1 time use)

1 Tbsp Apple Cider Vinegar
1 Cup warm water

(You can also add essential oils to give the ACV rinse mix some fragrance)

Directions

Mix the ACV and water in a small bottle. Shake the bottle. Apply the mix generously to your hair and scalp. Leave on your hair for about 2 minutes and then rinse out.

2. Aloe Vera Shampoo

Ingredients (for 1 time use)

3 Tbsp Aloe Vera Gel
4 Tbsp Coconut Milk
1 Tbsp Almond Oil

Directions

Add coconut milk, Aloe Vera gel and almond oil into a measuring jar or bowl. Use a wire whisk or spoon to mix until a thin consistency (takes about 30 to 35 seconds). Pour mix into a small bottle. Apply to hair and scalp, gently massaging scalp for a minute and then rinse out.

Conditioners

1. Mayonnaise Conditioner

Ingredients (for 1 time use)

½ cup mayonnaise
½ cup olive oil
2 egg yolks

Directions

Add egg yolks, mayonnaise and olive oil into a measuring jar or bowl. Use a wire whisk or spoon to mix until a thin consistency (takes about 1 minute). Pour mix into a bottle. Apply mix generously to damp hair, making sure not to forget the ends. Cover your hair with a plastic cap and let it sit for 30 minutes. Rinse out thoroughly.

2. Mayo and Avocado Conditioner

Ingredients (for 1 time use)

1 avocado

1 cup mayonnaise

2 Tbsp olive oil

Directions

Cut avocado in half and scoop out avocado flesh into a bowl. Add mayonnaise and oil. Mix well with a spoon or wire whisk until a creamy consistency. Apply mix generously to damp hair, making sure not to forget the ends. Cover with a plastic shower cap and let sit for 30 minutes. Rinse out thoroughly.

HOW TO MAKE YOUR OWN SHAMPOO AND CONDITIONER

RECOMMENDED HAIR TOOLKIT

For detangling:

Plastic wide tooth comb

Hercules Sagemann Magic Star Seamless Comb

Denman Classic styling brush

For styling:

Satin Scrunchies

Silk head ties

Bobby pins

For protecting your hair while you sleep:

Silk / satin scarf

Silk/ satin bonnet

Silk / satin pillow case

For drying after washing your hair:

Old T -shirt

Microfiber towel

Blow dryer (use on low to medium setting)

Hooded dryer (optional)

For daily moisturizing:

A spray bottle

For hot oil treatments:

Applicator bottle

For deep conditioning:

Plastic cap

Plastic grocery bag

Hooded dryer (optional)

For trimming your hair:

Hair shears

FINDING A GOOD HAIR STYLIST

Tips on finding a good hairstylist

1. *Use referrals.* Referrals are the best way to find a hairstylist. Ask friends, family or a stranger whose hairstyle you like. Be sure to let your new hairstylist know that you were referred and you were told she does a good job.

2. *Interest.* Make sure the hairstylist has interest in your hair and just doesn't see you as a walking cash dispenser.

3. *Interview the hairstylist.* Call ahead and ask when you can come in for few minutes to ask questions.

4. *Review sites.* Check out review sites (yelp.com, google.com reviews, angieslist.com).

5. *Be clear.* Be sure to be *very clear* with your hairstylist on what you want. If you want a trim, let them know exactly

how much length you want trimmed — don't go in saying you want a trim — you will end up getting more of a haircut. You are not being "bossy", you are speaking up for yourself.

6. *Male hairstylists.* Don't overlook male hairstylists, some of the best hairstylists in the world are male. Male hairstylists know that there is a gender bias and most will go out of their way to make you feel comfortable.

Always remember, a good hairstylist:

1. Will welcome your questions and answer them to your satisfaction.

2. Will keep her shop and workspace clean. If they don't take pride in the appearance of their workspace, how will they take pride in the appearance of their work?

3. Will not pressure you to do a certain hairstyle that is easier for her or a service that will pay her more. Don't give in to pressure from your hairstylist — you will regret it.

4. Will remember you are the customer and the customer is

Queen.

5. Will keep themselves updated on the latest trends and practices in hair care. Nothing worse than having a hair stylist who is stuck in her ways and is not willing to constantly educate herself.

6. Will not take an unreasonable amount of time doing your hair, while socializing or chatting on the phone.

INGREDIENTS TO LOOK FOR IN YOUR PRODUCTS

Water

Water moisturizes the hair. Our hair needs frequent hydration.

Vegetable glycerin / Glycerin

Vegetable glycerin is a by-product in the manufacture of vegetable oil. It is a humectant, helping to moisturize your hair.

Panthenol

Panthenol helps to moisturize your hair and is excellent for giving shine to the hair.

Collagen

Collagen is a protein and helps to strengthen your hair and reduce hair breakage.

Shea butter

Shea butter is both a humectant and an emollient. An

emollient is a substance that helps to soften the hair.

Wheat germ oil

Wheat germ oil has high amounts of Vitamin E which is good for your hair.

Coconut oil

Coconut oil is able to penetrate the cuticle and help in moisturizing your hair.

Aloe Vera

Aloe Vera helps in moisturizing the hair as a humectant.

Honey

Honey is a humectant and helps to moisturize your hair.

Tea tree oil

Tea tree oil has antifungal properties and is good in the prevention of dandruff.

Avocado oil

Avocado oil is a humectant and absorbs moisture from the air. Avocado oil also has protein which helps to strengthen hair.

Cocamidopropyl betaine

Cocamidopropyl betaine is a surfactant derived from coconut oil. It is commonly found in baby soaps and shampoos. It cleanses the hair and scalp without causing irritation.

Jojoba Oil

Jojoba Oil is an excellent sealant. Prevents moisture from being lost by the hair.

Stearyl Alcohol

Stearyl Alcohol is good for its smoothing properties and helps in moisturizing the hair.

Gentle Sulfates that are less drying to your hair:

Sodium Lauryl Sulfoacetate

Sodium Socoyl Sarcosinate

Sodium Cocyl Isethionate

Good Silicones:

Stearoxy Dimethicone

Behenoxy Dimethicone

INGREDIENTS TO LOOK FOR IN YOUR PRODUCTS

INGREDIENTS TO AVOID IN YOUR PRODUCTS

Parabens

Parabens are chemicals used in some shampoos and conditioners as preservatives. Some studies have found parabens in cancer patients and should be avoided if you can.

Petroleum / Petrolatum /Mineral Oils

Petroleum is a very common ingredient in black hair care products. While it is very effective as a sealant, it also prevents moisture absorption into the hair.

Alcohol / Isopropyl Alcohol

Alcohol / Isopropyl alcohol will dry your hair, which can lead to breakage.

Formaldehyde

Formaldehyde is a chemical preservative that kills bacteria. It is also a known carcinogen (cancer causing chemical) and has been known to cause allergic reactions. The main reason why it's used is because it is cheap. Avoid it if you can.

Harsh Sulfates that are drying to your hair:

Sodium Lauryl Sulfate (SLS)

 Sodium Laureth Sulfate (SLES)

 Sodium Olefin Sulfonate

Silicones that will cause build up easily:

Dimethicone

Cetyl Dimethicone

Cetearyl Methicone

GLOSSARY

A

APL

Arm Pit Length.

Active Ingredient

An ingredient with the highest concentration in a product. Usually listed first on the product ingredient label.

ACV

Apple Cider Vinegar.

Alopecia

General term used for hair loss.

Alopecia Androgenetic

Hair loss due to genetic predisposition.

Alopecia Areata
Hair loss in round patches, caused by genetic predisposition.

Alopecia Follicularis
Hair loss due to inflamed follicles.

Alopecia Senilis
Hair loss due to old age.

Alcohol
A common ingredient in hair products. Certain types of alcohol can be drying to the hair, while others add softness to the hair.

Alkaline
A substance when tested with a pH strip, has a pH greater than 7.

ALS
Ammonium Lauryl Sulfate.

Anagen

Anagen is the active growth phase of the hair growth cycle.

B

B5

Vitamin B5 also known as pantothenic acid.

Baggying

A technique used to moisturize the hair.

BC (same as Big Chop)

Is the single act of cutting off all your relaxed hair for the purpose of wearing your hair natural.

Bonding

A technique used to attach hair extensions.

Bulb

The base of the hair.

Braid out

A hair style that is also a protective style.

BSL

Bra Strap Length.

BSS

Beauty Supply Store.

Butyl Glycol

A chemical compound used as a conditioning agent.

C

Capillaries

Blood vessels that carry nutrients to your hair follicle.

Carrier Oil

Any oil used to dilute an essential oil. They "carry" an essential oil to the skin.

Carbomer

A gelling agent.

Catagen

Is the middle stage in the hair growth cycle, between the anagen and the telogen phases.

CBL

Collar Bone Length.

Cetyl Alcohol

An alcohol compound used as a conditioning agent and emollient.

Chelating Shampoo

A shampoo that is formulated to remove mineral deposits from the hair.

Clarifying Shampoo

A shampoo that is formulated to remove product build up and chlorine from the hair.

Coconut Oil

An oil good for smoothing and sealing the hair.

Conditioner

A creamy product often used after shampooing to improve the condition of the hair.

Co-Wash (Conditioner Wash or CW)

Using a conditioner to wash the hair.

Cone

Short for silicone.

Cortex

Middle layer of the hair strand.

Cream Rinse

Conditioner used for detangling.

Crown

Top of the hair.

Cuticle

Outer layer of the hair strand.

D

Dandruff

General term used for dead skin cells that have been shed from the scalp.

Dermal Papilla

Part of the hair follicle that supplies nutrients to the hair bulb.

Dermal Sheath

Lining around a hair strand.

Dermis

The middle layer of the skin that houses the blood vessels, the hair follicle and the sebaceous glands.

Deep Conditioning (also DC)

A method to condition the hair. The conditioner is left on the hair for a longer amount of time and then rinsed out.

Dimethicone

An ingredient used in a conditioner to aid detangling.

Diazolidnyl

A Chemical preservative.

Dreadlocks

A term for locks considered derogatory.

Dusting

A light trim.

E

Elasticity

The hairs ability to stretch and return to normal, without breaking.

Emollient

An ingredient that helps smooth or soften the hair.

Epidermis

The top layer of the skin.

Essential Oil

A natural oil usually obtained by distillation of a plant. It carries the "essence" of the plant.

EVCO

Extra Virgin Coconut Oil.

EVOO

Extra Virgin Olive Oil.

F

Follicle

An opening in the skin in which the hair grows out of.

Frizz

A condition of the hair when it clumps into tight curls caused by lack of moisture.

G

Glycerin

A by-product in the making of vegetable oil. Used as a humectant.

H

Henna

A vegetable dye prepared from the Henna plant.

HE

Herbal Essence.

HEHH

Herbal Essence Hello Hydration Conditioner. A very popular conditioner.

HL

Hip Length.

Humectant

Any substance that draws moisture from the air.

I

Isopropyl Lanolate

A synthetic moisturizer.

J

JBCO

Jamaican Black Castor Oil

Jojoba Oil

An oil good for smoothing and sealing the hair.

K

Keratin
Is a hard fibrous protein. The main component of hair and nails.

Kitchen
An area at the nape, considered the most difficult to keep straight when you have your hair relaxed.

L

Leave-in conditioner
A conditioner applied after washing the hair and left in the hair instead of being immediately rinsed out.

Length check
Measuring the length of the hair.

M

Matte

A non-shiny, dull look.

MBL

Mid Back Length.

Medulla

The inner most layer of the hair shaft.

Melanin

The body's natural pigment. Gives color to the skin and the hair.

Methylparaben

A chemical preservative.

Moisturizer

A product used to add moisture to the hair.

N

Natural

Not produced in a laboratory.

Natural hair

Hair that has not been chemically processed.

Neutralize

To reduce or negate. Commonly used in referring to reducing the pH level.

NG

New Growth.

NL

Neck Length.

No Poo

No shampoo method of washing the hair.

Nutrient

Any substance that provides nourishment for growth or metabolism .

O

Organic

Derived from plants.

Outer Root Sheath
A layer that surrounds the bottom of the hair strand.

P

Papilla

A part of the hair root that provides nutrients to the hair required for hair growth.

Panthenol

An ingredient that helps to moisturize and add shine to the hair.

Petroleum / Petrolatum

A common ingredient in Black hair products.

Permanent Color

A dye that is permanent and cannot be removed through washing.

PH

Percentage of hydrogen in a substance. It is a measure of the acidity or basicity of a solution.

PH Strip

A strip used to measure the pH level.

Pore

An opening of the sweat glands in the skin.

Porosity

The ability to absorb and retain moisture.

Pre Poo

A technique used to protect the hair from drying prior to shampooing.

Protein

A major component of hair.

Protein treatment

A hair care method used to add strength and temporarily repair damaged hair.

Propylene Glycol

A common ingredient in conditioners. Helps to moisturize the hair.

Propylparaben

A chemical preservative.

Protective Style

Any hairstyle that protects the hair ends from breakage.

R

Relaxer

A chemical used to straighten or loosen the natural curl pattern.

Remi/Remy Hair

High quality human hair that has cuticles intact and running in the same direction.

S

Scab hair

After a big chop, new growth that is dry and wiry. It is not the real texture of your hair. It caused by over processing when relaxing the hair.

Sealing

Method to lock in moisture in the hair. Done either by using an oil or a butter.

Sebaceous Gland
Gland in the skin whose job is to produce sebum, a natural lubricant.

Sebum
An oil produced by the sebaceous gland that lubricates the hair strand and scalp.

Sectioning
Dividing your hair into manageable areas when detangling, washing or conditioning. Usually done in 4 or more sections.

Semi Permanent Color
A color that will last 6 to 12 shampoo washes.

Serum
Smoothing product that keeps the hair from frizzing.

Silicone
A compound of silicon used to increase wet and dry compatibility.

Slip

Description for a conditioner that helps in the separation of hair strands and detangling.

SLS

Sodium Lauryl Sulfate.

Split Ends

The splitting or fraying of the hair.

Spritz

A hair spray.

Steaming

A method of moisturizing the hair using steam.

Stearic Acid / Stearyl Alcohol

An emollient that also helps in moisturizing the hair.

Stretching

Extending the length of time between relaxers.

SL

Shoulder Length.

Surfactants

In shampoos, a substance that allows oil and water to mix producing a lathering effect. Surfactants have a drying effect on your hair.

T

Telogen

Telogen is the resting phase of the hair growth cycle.

Temporary Color

A hair color that washes off after shampooing.

Texlaxing

A method of relaxing hair when the hair is intentionally under processed. Texlaxed hair has some thickness to it.

Texturizing

A method of relaxing hair which slightly relaxes the natural curl pattern.

Transitioning

The process of going from relaxed hair to natural hair.

Traction Alopecia

Hair loss due to the pulling of the hair.

Treatment

A hair care method used on a "as needed" basis. Done either to strengthen or to moisturize the hair.

TWA

Teeny Weeny Afro.

Twist Out

A popular hairstyle that is also a protective style.

V

Virgin Hair

Hair that is in its original state and has not been chemically processed.

W

WL

Waist Length.

To order additional copies or discounts on
bulk orders please visit
www.theblackhairbible.com